Clinical Focus on
Endometriosis

Clinical Focus on
Endometriosis

Series Editors

Neharika Malhotra
MD (Gold Medalist) DRM (Germany) FICMCH Fellow
ICOG (Rep Med) ICOG (USG)
Director and Consultant
ART Rainbow IVF and MNMH (P) Ltd
and Ujala Cygnus Rainbow Hospital
Agra, Uttar Pradesh, India
Joint Secretary, FOGSI
Chair, YTP Committee, FOGSI

Jaideep Malhotra
MD FICMCH FICOG FRCOG FRCPI FMAS
Managing Director
ART Rainbow IVF and MNMH (P) Ltd
and Ujala Cygnus Rainbow Hospital
Agra, Uttar Pradesh, India
President, SAFOM/ISPAT
Past President, IMS/ISAR/FOGSI/ASPIRE

Narendra Malhotra
MD FICMCH FICOG FRCOG FICS FMAS FIAP
Managing Director
Global Rainbow Health Care and MNMH (P) Ltd
and Ujala Cygnus Rainbow Hospital
Agra, Uttar Pradesh, India
Professor, Sarajevo School of Science and Technology, Croatia
Past President, FOGSI/IFUMB/ISPAT/ISAR, INSARG
Vice President, WAPM/SAFOG
Director, International IAN Donald School and SAFOG

Editors

Aruna Suman
MD FICOG
Professor and Head
Department of Obstetrics and Gynecology
Government Medical College
Hyderabad, Telangana, India

Panchampreet Kaur
DGO DNB MNAMS FICMCH
Assistant Professor
Obstetrics and Gynecology
Lady Hardinge Medical College and Smt SK Hospital
New Delhi, India

Rohan Palshetkar
MS (Obs and Gyne) FRM BDRME ADRME
Associate Professor
Head of Unit Bloom IVF
Mumbai, Maharashtra, India

Kalyan B Barmade
DNB FCPS DGO DFP
Consultant, Gynec Endoscopic Surgeon and IVF Specialists
Director, Department of Obstetrics and Gynecology
Latur Fertility Center Pvt Ltd
Latur, Maharashtra, India

Foreword
Nandita Palshetkar

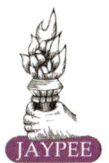

JAYPEE BROTHERS MEDICAL PUBLISHERS
The Health Sciences Publisher
New Delhi | London

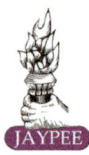
Jaypee Brothers Medical Publishers (P) Ltd.

Headquarters
Jaypee Brothers Medical Publishers (P) Ltd
EMCA House, 23/23-B
Ansari Road, Daryaganj
New Delhi 110 002, India
Landline: +91-11-23272143, +91-11-23272703
+91-11-23282021, +91-11-23245672
Email: jaypee@jaypeebrothers.com

Corporate Office
Jaypee Brothers Medical Publishers (P) Ltd
4838/24, Ansari Road, Daryaganj
New Delhi 110 002, India
Phone: +91-11-43574357
Fax: +91-11-43574314
Email: jaypee@jaypeebrothers.com

Overseas Office
JP Medical Ltd.
83, Victoria Street, London
SW1H 0HW (UK)
Phone: +44 20 3170 8910
Fax: +44 (0)20 3008 6180
Email: info@jpmedpub.com

Website: www.jaypeebrothers.com
Website: www.jaypeedigital.com

© 2024, Jaypee Brothers Medical Publishers

The views and opinions expressed in this book are solely those of the original contributor(s)/author(s) and do not necessarily represent those of editor(s) or publisher of the book.

All rights reserved. No part of this publication may be reproduced, stored or transmitted in any form or by any means, electronic, mechanical, photocopying, recording or otherwise, without the prior permission in writing of the publishers.

All brand names and product names used in this book are trade names, service marks, trademarks or registered trademarks of their respective owners. The publisher is not associated with any product or vendor mentioned in this book.

Medical knowledge and practice change constantly. This book is designed to provide accurate, authoritative information about the subject matter in question. However, readers are advised to check the most current information available on procedures included and check information from the manufacturer of each product to be administered, to verify the recommended dose, formula, method and duration of administration, adverse effects and contraindications. It is the responsibility of the practitioner to take all appropriate safety precautions. Neither the publisher nor the author(s)/editor(s) assume any liability for any injury and/or damage to persons or property arising from or related to use of material in this book.

This book is sold on the understanding that the publisher is not engaged in providing professional medical services. If such advice or services are required, the services of a competent medical professional should be sought.

Every effort has been made where necessary to contact holders of copyright to obtain permission to reproduce copyright material. If any have been inadvertently overlooked, the publisher will be pleased to make the necessary arrangements at the first opportunity.

Inquiries for bulk sales may be solicited at: jaypee@jaypeebrothers.com

Clinical Focus on Endometriosis

First Edition: **2024**

ISBN: 978-93-5696-126-5

Printed at: Replika Press Pvt. Ltd.

Dedicated to

Our parents, teachers, and all practicing obstetricians and gynecologists

Contributors

Aarti Chitkara Wadhawan
MBBS MD (PGI, Chandigarh)
ICOG Fellow: Gynecology Endoscopy
Senior Resident
Department of Obstetrics and Gynecology
All India Institute of Medical Sciences
New Delhi, India

Anand B Barmade
MD (Medicine) FRCGP
Family Physician
Department of General Physician
Parkgate Medical Centre
South Yorkshire, England, UK

Ankita Bansal Goyal
MD (PGIMER, CHD) DNB MRCOG
Consultant
Sankalp Hospital
Department of Obstetrics and Gynecology
Ambikapur, Chhattisgarh, India

Aruna Suman MD FICOG
Professor and Head
Department of Obstetrics and Gynecology
Government Medical College
Hyderabad, Telangana, India

C Archana Devi
MD MRCOG
Consultant
Department of Obstetrics and Gynecology
Ramakrishna Medical Center LLP
Trichy, Tamil Nadu, India

Jaideep Malhotra
MD FICMCH FICOG FRCOG FRCPI FMAS
Managing Director
ART Rainbow IVF and MNMH (P) Ltd
and Ujala Cygnus Rainbow Hospital
Agra, Uttar Pradesh, India
President, SAFOM/ISPAT
Past President, IMS/ISAR/FOGSI/ASPIRE

Kalyan B Barmade DNB FCPS DGO DFP
Consultant
Gynec Endoscopic Surgeon and IVF Specialists
Director
Department of Obstetrics and Gynecology
Latur Fertility Center Pvt Ltd
Latur, Maharashtra, India

Manisha K Barmade MBBS DGO
Consultant and Director
Department of Obstetrics and Gynecology
Latur Fertility Center Pvt Ltd
Latur, Maharashtra, India

Manisha Nandi MS
Reproductive Medicine Fellow
Department of Reproductive Medicine
Bloom IVF
Mumbai, Maharashtra, India

Mayuri More MS FRM
Assistant Professor
Department of Obstetrics and Gynecology
DY Patil School of Medicine
Mumbai, Maharashtra, India

Monisha Singh MBBS MD (Obs-Gyn)
Consultant
Department of Obstetrics and Gynecology
Parul Hospital and Sarojini Hospital
Varanasi, Uttar Pradesh, India

Narendra Malhotra
MD FICMCH FICOG FRCOG FICS FMAS FIAP
Managing Director
Global Rainbow Health Care and MNMH (P) Ltd
and Ujala Cygnus Rainbow Hospital
Agra, Uttar Pradesh, India
Professor, Sarajevo School of Science and Technology, Croatia
Past President, FOGSI/IFUMB/ISPAT/ISAR, INSARG
Vice President, WAPM/SAFOG
Director, International IAN Donald School and SAFOG

Neharika Malhotra
MD (Gold Medalist) DRM (Germany) FICMCH Fellow
ICOG (Rep Med) ICOG (USG)
Director and Consultant
ART Rainbow IVF and MNMH (P) Ltd
and Ujala Cygnus Rainbow Hospital
Agra, Uttar Pradesh, India
Joint Secretary, FOGSI
Chair, YTP Committee, FOGSI

Panchampreet Kaur
DGO DNB MNAMS FICMCH
Assistant Professor
Obstetrics and Gynecology
Lady Hardinge Medical College and
Smt SK Hospital
New Delhi, India

Ritu Hinduja
MD MRM (UK) DRM (Germany) FICOG Fellowship
in Reproductive Medicine (India, Spain, Israel)
Certificate in Genetic Counseling
Cluster Head and Senior Consultant
Fertility Specialist, NOVA IVF Fertility
Mumbai, Maharashtra, India

Rohan Palshetkar
MS (Obs and Gyne) FRM BDRME ADRME
Associate Professor
Head of Unit Bloom IVF
Mumbai, Maharashtra, India

T Ramani Devi MD DGO FICS FICOG
Director and Consultant
Department of Obstetrics and Gynecology
Ramakrishna Medical Center LLP and
Janani Fertility Center
Trichy, Tamil Nadu, India

Foreword

Dear Readers,

Endometriosis is a condition that affects millions of individuals around the world, yet it remains widely misunderstood and often overlooked. As a gynecologist who has treated thousands of cases of endometriosis it is a pleasure to see the Series Editors Dr Neharika Malhotra, Dr Jaideep Malhotra, and Dr Narendra Malhotra along with the Editors of this book, Dr Aruna Suman, Dr Panchampreet Kaur, Dr Rohan Palshetkar, and Dr Kalyan B Barmade release this Endometriosis Focus.

As someone who has personally witnessed the physical and emotional toll that endometriosis can take on individuals, I am deeply grateful for the dedication and passion of the authors in bringing this book to life. Their commitment to raising awareness and offering guidance is evident on every page.

You will find a comprehensive exploration of endometriosis, from its mysterious origins to the latest advancements in diagnosis and treatment. The authors have put in extensive research and come with latest advances to update you with current trends in the management of endometriosis. This book provides a wealth of knowledge and I am sure you are going to have a fantastic read.

The book is going to be an in-depth dive into the challenges that we face in endometriosis and a call to action for all of us to work together in eliminating this enigmatic disease. I hope this book helps you in your day-to-day practice and you are able to apply the knowledge you gain to better the care you can provide to your patients.

Happy reading

Nandita Palshetkar
MD DGO FCPS FICOG FRCOG
Medical Director, Bloom IVF-India
Mumbai, Maharashtra, India
President, ISAR (2022–24)
Past President, FOGSI, IAGE, AMOGS, MOGS
FOGSI Representative to FIGO

Preface

The editors of this *Clinical Focus on Endometriosis* have worked hard to get a ready-reckoner for all practicing obstetricians and gynecologists. This book is a compilation of chapters to help the readers manage endometriosis easily and confidently. Each chapter has been immaculately formulated to present working knowledge of the latest management protocols. The chapter contributors have put the complex problem of endometriosis in simple format which can be read easily and understood by all. We sincerely hope that the readers will find this book very useful to students, teachers, and practitioners.

"Reading is the gateway skill the makes all other learning possible."

Neharika Malhotra
Jaideep Malhotra
Narendra Malhotra

Acknowledgments

We have the pleasure of introducing *Clinical Focus on Endometriosis*.

We thank the Almighty God for helping us throughout the journey of completing this task. Our heartfelt gratitude to Dr Nandita Palshetkar for accepting to write the foreword for this book and also give her blessings.

It is with utmost pleasure that we thank Dr Narendra Malhotra, Dr Jaideep Malhotra and Dr Neharika Malhotra, our mentors and guide for this clinical series, who lent their considerable clinical and academic prowess.

We wish to thank all our contributors who responded to our requests with promptness. Our heartfelt thanks to them. We wish to appreciate the efforts of M/s Jaypee Brothers Medical Publishers (P) Ltd, New Delhi, India for bringing out this book in its final shape with their talent of skillfully and expediently coordinating and overseeing composition. We also thank publishing team of M/s Jaypee Brothers Medical Publishers, especially Ms Pallavi A Mehrotra. Without the thoughtful, creative efforts of many, our Focus Series would have been a barren wasteland of words. Their attention to detail and accurate renderings added important academic support to our words.

Our special appreciation and thanks to all our colleagues and friends who supported our idea of bringing out this series and gave us the confidence to finish this book. Lastly, we offer an enthusiastic thanks to our families and friends. We sincerely thank you for your love and support which kept us going to finish this work of ours.

Aruna Suman
Panchampreet Kaur
Rohan Palshetkar
Kalyan B Barmade

Contents

1. **Endometriosis an Enigma, a Benign Cancer: An Epiphenomenon** 1
   Aarti Chitkara Wadhawan, Narendra Malhotra, Neharika Malhotra

2. **Newer Thoughts on Etiopathology, Staging, and Guidelines** 6
   Panchampreet Kaur, Jaideep Malhotra, Neharika Malhotra

3. **Clinical Presentation: Endometriosis** 15
   Kalyan B Barmade, Manisha K Barmade

4. **Diagnosis of Endometriosis** 17
   Aruna Suman, Panchampreet Kaur

5. **Endometriosis Scoring Systems** 24
   Monisha Singh, Narendra Malhotra, Neharika Malhotra, Jaideep Malhotra

6. **Medical Management of Endometriosis** 36
   Kalyan B Barmade, Manisha K Barmade, Anand B Barmade

7. **Surgical Management of Endometriosis** 40
   Ankita Bansal Goyal, Aruna Suman

8. **Endometriosis and Assisted Reproduction Technology** 44
   T Ramani Devi, C Archana Devi

9. **Future and Stem Cell Therapy** 57
   Kalyan B Barmade, Manisha K Barmade, Anand B Barmade

10. **Endometriosis and Intrauterine Insemination Protocols** 60
    Rohan Palshetkar, Manisha Nandi

11. **Endometriosis and In Vitro Fertilization** 67
    Rohan Palshetkar, Mayuri More, Manisha Nandi

12. **Recurrent Endometriosis** 75
    Rohan Palshetkar, Ritu Hinduja

Index 83

CHAPTER 1

Endometriosis an Enigma, a Benign Cancer: An Epiphenomenon

Aarti Chitkara Wadhawan, Narendra Malhotra, Neharika Malhotra

INTRODUCTION

Endometriosis is a common disease in women, causing pelvic pain and infertility. It is characterized by the presence of endometrial tissue, composed of epithelial glands and endometrial stromal cells, outside the uterus. It is an extremely heterogenous clinical entity with regard to etiopathogenesis, clinical features, and treatment.

Although benign, endometriosis has cancer-like features, a mutation profile similar to that of an ovarian cancer (OC), and an increased risk of OC.[1-3] They result in local and distant metastasis, invasion and destruction of adjacent structures, unrestricted growth, resistance to apoptosis, development of new blood vessels, etc.

The lifetime risk of OC among women with endometriosis is 1.80%, fewer than 2 women in 100,[4,5] thereby suggesting a very low overall risk of developing OC.

MECHANISM OF MALIGNANT TRANSFORMATION OF ENDOMETRIOSIS

Sampson in 1925[6] proposed three criteria for the diagnosis of endometriosis-associated OC (EOAC):
1. Evidence of endometriosis close to the tumor
2. Exclusion of invasion from other sources
3. Presence of tissue resembling endometrial stroma surrounding characteristic epithelial glands.

Scott in 1953[7] revised the criteria and added the fourth criterion:
4. Histological proof of transitions from benign changes in endometriosis to malignant changes.

Endometriosis is associated with genetic instability and several genetic alterations. Few mutations shared by both endometriosis and endometriosis-associated malignancy (EAM) are loss of heterozygosity at 10q23, PTEN (phosphatase and tensin homolog deleted on chromosome 10), ARID1A (AT-rich interactive domain-containing protein 1A), and p53 mutations.[8]

A proposed mechanism of pathway postulated for EAM is depicted in **Flowchart 1**.

Two potential mechanisms leading to EOAC have been proposed:
1. Extracellular hemoglobin, iron, and heme (from the repeated hemorrhages occurring in the endometriosis) causing cellular oxidative damage via increased reactive oxygen species with subsequent deoxyribonucleic acid (DNA) damage and resulting mutations
2. The second mechanism involves persistent production of antioxidants, which would favor a tumor-potentiating environment.

Flowchart 1: Mechanism of malignant transformation in endometriosis.

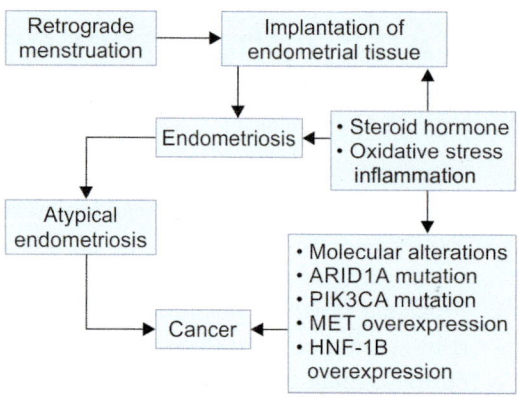

Flowchart 2: Potential process of the establishment and evolution of endometriosis lesions to ovarian cancer.

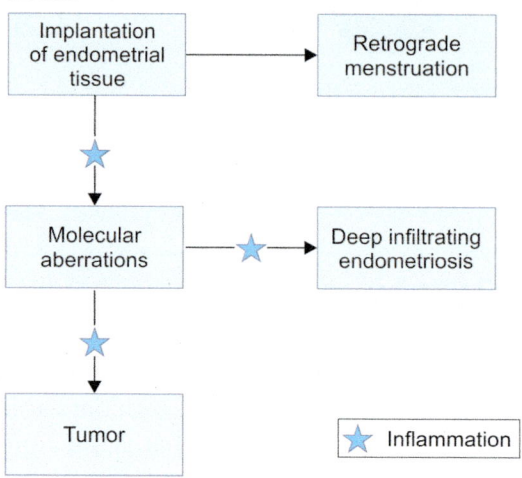

(ARID1A: AT-rich interactive domain-containing protein 1A; HNF-1B: hepatocyte nuclear factor 1-beta; MET: mesenchymal-epithelial transition factor; PIK3CA: phosphatidylinositol-4, 5-bisphosphate 3-kinase catalytic subunit alpha)

Both of these result in a double-edged sword redox imbalance milieu.[9,10]

Flowchart 2 illustrates the potential process of establishment and evolution of endometriosis lesions to ovarian cancer.

Risk factors that lead to transformation of endometriosis from benign to borderline (atypical) and then to EOAC involve molecular genomic alteration, inflammation, hyperestrogenism, oxidative stress, and obesity. Molecular alterations such as mutations of ARID1A, PI3KCA (phosphoinositide 3-kinases), loss of heterozygosity of PTEN, HNF-1b (hepatocyte nuclear factor-1b), and mutation of CTNNb1 (catenin beta 1) are illustrated in **Flowchart 3**.[11]

Endometroid and clear cell carcinoma are the most common types of ovarian carcinoma of EAOC with an incidence of 32% and 28%, respectively. Other less common types of malignancies encountered are the endocervical type of mucinous borderline tumor, endometrial stromal sarcoma, and Mullerian adenosarcoma.[12,13]

Flowchart 3: Molecular pathways involved in endometriosis-associated ovarian cancer pathogenesis.

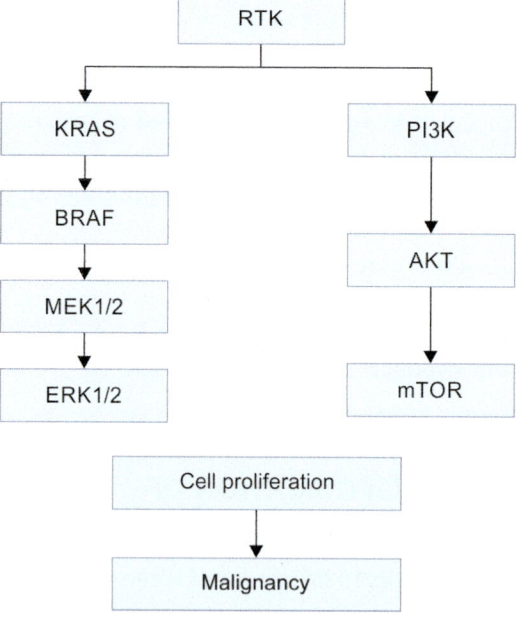

(AKT: AK strain transforming protein; BRAF: ERK 1/2: extracellular signal-regulated kinases; KRAS: Kirsten rat sarcoma viral oncogene homolog; MEK 1/2: mTOR: mammalian target of rapamycin; RTK: receptor tyrosine kinases)

The diagnostic dilemma between endometriosis and OC is further perplexed by raised cancer antigen (CA)-125 in both the entities. Human epididymis protein 4 (HE4) is a useful differentiating tumor marker, specifically for ovarian malignancy.

■ STEM CELLS

Some recent suggestions propose that endometriotic lesions originate from ectopic endometrial stem cell progenitors. This is supported by the fact that some Hox genes are involved in both eutopic endometrium and OC.[14-17] However, research in this area is far from offering any direct evidence; therefore, we can only hypothesize about the possible role of stem cells, and the calls of direct targeting as a therapeutical tool are yet to be established.

■ DIAGNOSIS

Early detection of malignant transformation is of paramount importance to improve the prognosis of EOAC. One should be cautious in women diagnosed with endometriosis at an early age, long-standing history, large endometrioma, and endometriosis-associated infertility.

With advancement in ultrasound and rising expertise in detecting subtle features on ultrasound, this can be a useful modality to diagnose early features of a malignant transformation of endometriosis. A unilocular cyst with papillary projection without ascites has been detected in most instances of EAOC in a multicenter study involving 239 women on ultrasound.[18] On T1-weighted images of contrast-enhanced magnetic resonance imaging (MRI), unilateral cystic mass containing hemorrhagic fluid and mural nodule is characteristic of malignant transformation of endometrioma. The disappearance of shading on T2-weighted images with enlargement of endometrioma is suggestive of malignant transformation.[19]

■ MANAGEMENT AND PROGNOSIS

Many experts observed a better prognosis compared with non-EOAC probably due to early stage and grade of the disease.[20] In a large population-based cohort study, longer survival was observed in OC patients with histologically proven endometriosis than those without endometriosis even after adjusting stage, grade, type, age at diagnosis, treatment protocol, and residual tumor after surgery.[21]

A recent meta-analysis demonstrated that EOAC patients had better overall survival (OS) as compared to non-EOAC patients in both OC and ovarian clear cell cancer (OCCC) cohorts. The meta-analysis also found that EOAC patients had better progression-free survival (PFS) than non-EOAC patients.[22]

■ ENDOMETRIOSIS AND OTHER MALIGNANCIES

A Swedish study of over 64,000 women found that patients with endometriosis have an increased risk of certain malignancies (ovarian, endocrine, non-Hodgkin lymphoma, and brain tumors), and this risk increases with early diagnosed or long-standing disease.[23] A study of 45,000 Danish women confirmed not only the increased risk of OC, but also the increased risks of endometrial and breast cancers.[24] In addition, the risk of colorectal cancer was increased 13-fold in women with internal endometriosis.[25]

■ PREVENTION

Studies are underway to identify specific biomarkers to identify endometriosis with oncogenic potential where specific targeted therapy can be offered. It has been observed that the risk of EOAC results in a 20–30% reduction with 5 years of use of oral contraceptives.[26]

No clear evidence exists that transvaginal ultrasound or CA-125 measurements can detect OCs early or that risk-reducing salpingo-oophorectomy can save lives. Generally, to improve health and reduce the risk of cancer, a balanced diet with a low intake of alcohol, regular exercise, healthy weight, and refraining from smoking is advisable.

■ CONCLUSION

There appears to be an increased risk of OC, particularly endometrioid and clear cell types, in individuals with ovarian endometriosis but not in patients with peritoneal or deeply infiltrating endometriosis. Some ovarian endometriosis lesions harbor genetic mutations in ARID1A, PTEN, HNF-1b and K-Ras that may also be found in ovarian cancer lesions. Future molecular analysis of surgical ovarian endometriosis specimens may help to identify patients at the highest risk of developing OC. While the relative risk of OC may be increased, the absolute risk of developing OC from ovarian endometriosis remains low, with approximately two additional cases per 10,000 women-years of follow-up for individuals with ovarian endometriosis compared with those without endometriosis.[27]

■ REFERENCES

1. Garry R. Endometriosis: an invasive disease. Gynaecol Endos. 2001;10(2):79-82.
2. Anglesio MS, Papadopoulos N, Ayhan A, Nazeran TM, Noë M, Horlings HM, et al. Cancer-associated mutations in endometriosis without cancer. N Engl J Med. 2017;376(19):1835-48.
3. Kvaskoff M, Mu F, Terry KL, Harris HR, Poole EM, Farland L, et al. Endometriosis: a high-risk population for major chronic diseases? Hum Reprod Update. 2015;21(4):500-16.
4. Kim HS, Kim TH, Chung HH, Song YS. Risk and prognosis of ovarian cancer in women with endometriosis: A meta-analysis. Br J Cancer. 2014;110(7):1878-90.
5. Wang C, Liang Z, Liu X, Zhang Q, Li S. The association between endometriosis, tubal ligation, hysterectomy and epithelial ovarian cancer: Meta-analyses. Int J Environ Res Public Health. 2016;13(11):1138.
6. Sampson JA. Endometrial carcinoma of the ovary, arising in endometrial tissue in that organ. Arch Surg. 1925;10(1):1-72.
7. Scott RB. Malignant changes in endometriosis. Obstet Gynecol. 1953;2(3):283-9.
8. Pollacco J, Sacco K, Portelli M, Schembri-Wismayer P, Calleja-Agius J. Molecular links between endometriosis and cancer. Gynecol Endocrinol. 2012;28(8):577-81.
9. Kobayashi H. Potential scenarios leading to ovarian cancer arising from endometriosis. Redox Rep. 2016;21(3):119-26.
10. Fontana J, Zima M, Vetvicka V. Biological markers of oxidative stress in cardiovascular diseases: after so many studies, what do we know? Immunol Invest. 2018;47(8):823-43.
11. Kurman RJ, Carcangiu ML, Herrington CS. WHO Classification of Tumours of the Female Reproductive Organs, 4th edition. Geneva: International Agency for Research on Cancer; 2014.
12. Krawczyk N, Banys-Paluchowski M, Schmidt D, Ulrich U, Fehm T. Endometriosis-associated malignancy. Geburtshilfe Frauenheilkd. 2016;76(2):176-81.
13. Nezhat F, Datta MS, Hanson V, Pejovic T, Nezhat C, Nezhat C. The relationship of endometriosis and ovarian malignancy: a review. Fertil Steril. 2008;90(5):1559-70.
14. Maruyama T, Yoshimura Y. Stem cell theory for the pathogenesis of endometriosis. Front Biosci (Elite Ed). 2012;4(8):2754-63.
15. Laganà AS, Vitale SG, Salmeri FM, Triolo O, Frangež HB, Vrtačnik-Bokal E, et al. Unus pro omnibus, omnes pro uno: a novel, evidence-based, unifying theory for the pathogenesis of endometriosis. Med Hypotheses. 2017;103:10-20

16. Laganà AS, Salmeri FM, Vitale SG, Triolo O, Götte M. Stem cell trafficking during endometriosis: may epigenetics play a pivotal role? Reprod Sci. 2018;25(7):978-9.
17. Cheng W, Liu J, Yoshida H, Rosen D, Naora H. Lineage infidelity of epithelial ovarian cancers is controlled by HOX genes that specify regional identity in the reproductive tract. Nat Med. 2005;11(5):531-7.
18. Moro F, Magoga G, Pasciuto T, Mascilini F, Moruzzi MC, Fischerova D, et al. Imaging in gynecological disease (13): clinical and ultrasound characteristics of endometrioid ovarian cancer. Ultrasound Obstet Gynecol. 2018;52(4):535-43.
19. Takeuchi M, Matsuzaki K, Uehara H, Nishitani H. Malignant transformation of pelvic endometriosis: MR imaging findings and pathologic correlation. Radiographics. 2006;26(2):407-17.
20. Kvaskoff M, Horne AW, Missmer SA. Informing women with endometriosis about ovarian cancer risk. Lancet. 2017;390(10111):2433-4
21. Hermens M, van Altena AM, Nieboer TE, Schoot BC, van Vliet HA, Siebers AG, et al. Incidence of endometrioid and clear-cell ovarian cancer in histological proven endometriosis: The ENOCA population-based cohort study. Am J Obstet Gynecol. 2020;223(1):107.e1-107.e11.
22. Chen P, Zhang CY. Association between endometriosis and prognosis of ovarian cancer: An updated meta-analysis. Front Oncol. 2022;12:732322.
23. Melin A, Sparen P, Persson I, Bergqvist A. Endometriosis and the risk of cancer with special emphasis on ovarian cancer. Human reproduction. Hum Reprod. 2006;21(5):1237-42.
24. Mogensen JB, Kjær SK, Mellemkjær L, Jensen A. Endometriosis and risks for ovarian, endometrial and breast cancers: a nationwide cohort study. Gynecol Oncol. 2016;143(1):87-92.
25. Kok VC, Tsai HJ, Su CF, Lee CK. The risks for ovarian, endometrial, breast, colorectal, and other cancers in women with newly diagnosed endometriosis or adenomyosis: a population-based study. Int J Gynecol Cancer. 2015;25(6):968-76.
26. Beral V, Doll R, Hermon C, Peto R, Reeves G. Ovarian cancer and oral contraceptives: collaborative reanalysis of data from 45 epidemiological studies including 23,257 women with ovarian cancer and 87,303 controls. Lancet. 2008;371(9609):303-14.
27. Saavalainen L, Lassus H, But A, Tiitinen A, Härkki P, Gissler M, et al. Risk of gynecologic cancer according to the type of endometriosis. Obstet Gynecol. 2018;131(6):1095-102.

Newer Thoughts on Etiopathology, Staging, and Guidelines

Panchampreet Kaur, Jaideep Malhotra, Neharika Malhotra

■ INTRODUCTION

Endometriosis is an inflammatory disease of chronic nature and involves the presence of endometrium-like tissue outside the uterus.[1,2] It presents most commonly as ovarian endometriotic cysts followed by extraovarian deposits in pouch of Douglas, peritoneum, bladder and rarely pleural and stomach deposits. The International Working Group of American Association of Gynecologic Laparoscopists (AAGL), European Society for Gynaecological Endoscopy (ESGE), European Society of Human Reproduction and Embryology (ESHRE), and World Endometriosis Society (WES), et al. have defined endometriosis as a disease characterized by the presence of endometrium-like epithelium and/or stroma outside the endometrium and myometrium, usually with an associated inflammatory process.[3] It generally affects 2–10% of women of reproductive age.[4]

■ ETIOPATHOGENESIS

Various theories which have been proposed that explain the origin and development of endometriosis are described hereunder.

Sampson's Theory of Retrograde Menstruation

This is the most common explanation theory which still holds its importance. It has been postulated that during menses, endometrial cells grow retrograde into the peritoneal cavity through the fallopian tubes and thereby get implanted there.[5] This theory is somewhat supported by the fact that incidence of endometriosis is increased in girls having obstructive müllerian anomalies. On the flip side, it has also been reported that not all who have retrograde menstruation will definitely have evidence of endometriosis.[6]

Premenarchal Endometriosis

There have been isolated reports of endometriosis in premenarchal girls which puts a jolt at the retrograde theory of menstruation as these girls present with endometriosis even before the menstruation starts.[7] The possible explanation supporting this includes the presence of müllerian embryonic rests and also neonatal uterine bleeding due to withdrawal of maternal hormones.

Microembolization

Spread of endometrial tissue in microemboli form through the venous or the lymphatics to distant organs like lungs is also a proposed theory. These microemboli are thought to affect both the hemithoraces equally although right side hemithorax has been seen to be involved in >80% of the patients.[8]

Coelomic Metaplasia

It has been proposed that pluripotent cells transform to differentiated endometrium and this theory has been supported by literature which reports a case of endometriosis in a young woman with Mayer-Rokitansky-Küster-Hauser syndrome.[9]

Genetics: Recently, genetic studies have identified genomic regions and abnormalities in cancer driver genes (*PIK3CA, KRAS, ARID1A*) associated with endometriosis.[10-12]

The gross endometriotic lesions have been categorically divided as superficial, deep, and ovarian.

Superficial peritoneal: These lesions or deposits can present superficially as peritoneal deposits. On histopathology, presence of endometrial glands and/or stroma is diagnostic of same. Occasionally, hormonal and metaplastic changes may mask the glandular component.

Deep endometriosis: Deep endometriosis is defined as presence of endometriotic deposits or tissue extending beneath the peritoneum. It is defined as lesion involving > 5 mm of depth into the peritoneum.[13] It is generally found in the ureter, bladder, rectosigmoid colon, rectum, rectovaginal septum and other pelvic tissues such as parametrium and vagina.

Ovarian endometriosis: It may present in the form of ovarian cysts of varying sizes. Endometriotic cyst can be confused with hemorrhagic cyst/corpus luteal cyst. Symptomatology of the patient and a repeat follow-up scan in postmenstrual phase can distinguish between the two. The physiology revolves around cyclical bleeding in the ectopic endometrial tissue at ovarian site resulting in a hemorrhagic collection over a period of time surrounded by ovarian parenchyma.[14]

The pain associated with endometriosis is usually due to inflammation and pain mediators in addition to some neurologic dysfunction. Endometriosis is associated with subfertility which may be the result of pelvic adhesions and anatomic distortion due to endometriotic cysts. The chemical milieu involving secretion of prostanoids, cytokines, and growth factors which are found in endometriosis might be antagonistic to gamete formation, sperm mobility, and fertilization process.

STAGING SYSTEMS AND GUIDELINES

Various classification systems have been reviewed. Classifying endometriosis helps overcoming the interobserver bias and corroborates the clinical and surgical findings thereby improving the treatment approach. This is helpful for research purposes as well. The standard systems which are usually considered include the revised American Society for Reproductive Medicine (rASRM) classification, Enzian classification, endometriosis fertility index (EFI), and AAGL classification. The WES has given guidance to use rASRM classification, Enzian classification (in case of deep infiltrating endometriosis) and EFI classification (in cases of desired future fertility) for a comprehensive approach and further treatment.

The American Society for Reproductive Medicine Revised Classification[15]

The rASRM classification has been depicted in **Table 1** and comprises following stages.

Stage 1 (Minimal)

Score 1–5: Superficial peritoneal and ovarian implants and filmy adhesions in one or both ovaries.

TABLE 1: American Society for Reproductive Medicine (ASRM) revised classification of endometriosis.[15]

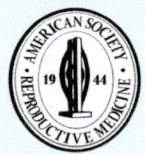

Patient's name_____ Date_____

Stage I (Minimal) — 1–5
Stage II (Mild) — 6–15
Stage III (Moderate) — 16–40
Stage IV (Severe) — >40
Total_____

Laparoscopy_____ Laparotomy_____ Photography_____
Recommended treatment_____
_____
Prognosis_____
_____

	Endometriosis	<1 cm	1–3 cm	>3 cm
Peritoneum	Superficial	1	2	4
	Deep	2	4	6
Ovary	R Superficial	1	2	4
	Deep	4	16	20
	L Superficial	1	2	4
	Deep	4	16	20
	Posterior cul-de-sac obliteration	Partial		Complete
		4		40
	Adhesions	<1/3 enclosure	1/3–2/3 enclosure	>2/3 enclosure
Ovary	R Filmy	1	2	4
	Dense	4	8	16
	L Filmy	1	2	4
	Dense	4	8	16
Tube	R Filmy	1	2	4
	Dense	4*	8*	16
	L Filmy	1	2	4
	Dense	4*	8*	16

*If the fimbriated end of the fallopian tube is completely enclosed, change the point assignment to 16.
Denote appearance of superficial implant types as red [(R), red, red-pink, flamelike, vesicular blobs, clear vesicles], white [(W), opacifications, peritoneal defects, yellow-brown], or black [(B), black, hemosiderin deposits, blue]. Denote percent of total described as R___%, W___% and B___%. Total should equal 100%.

Stage 2 (Mild)

Score 6-15: Few superficial and a few deep implants in the peritoneum and ovaries, filmy adhesions, and small chocolate cysts in the ovaries.

Stage 3 (Moderate)

Score 16-40: Deep peritoneal implants, ovarian cysts, dense tubal adhesions and/or partial posterior cul-de-sac obliteration.

Stage 4 (Severe)

Score >40: Many deep peritoneal implants, large chocolate cysts, many dense adhesions, and complete cul-de-sac obliteration.

The rASRM score does not consider the deep infiltrating endometriosis involving the retroperitoneal structures and there is a weak correlation between the extent of endometriosis and pain, sterility, and surgical complexity. So, newer classifications were made. Adamson and Pasta described the EFI classification in 2010 which considered the clinical and the surgical factors **(Tables 2 to 4)**.[16]

The Enzian classification was developed in 2005 in Austria[17] due to paucity of description on deeply infiltrating endometriosis in the previous classifications. The same was revised in 2011 for better comprehension.

Revised Enzian Classification

They have divided structures into various compartments. Retroperitoneal structures are categorized into the following three compartments: Compartment A includes vaginal and rectovaginal septum (RVS), compartment B has uterosacral ligament up to pelvic wall and compartment C for rectum and sigmoid colon. Severity is graded from grades 1 to 3 which are defined as invasion < 1 cm, 1–3 cm, and > 3 cm, respectively. If there are several foci, then the largest focus in each compartment is evaluated.

Deep invasion of endometriosis beyond the lesser pelvis in distant sites can be described separately and is labeled as prefix "F" which stands for "far" or "foreign," [FA = adenomyosis, FB = involvement of the bladder, FU = intrinsic involvement of the ureter,

TABLE 2: Terminology used in endometriosis fertility index (EFI) classification.[16]

Structure	Dysfunction	Description
Tube	Mild	Slight injury to tubal serosa
	Moderate	Moderate injury to serosa or muscularis layer of the fallopian tube, moderate limitation in mobility
	Severe	Fallopian tube fibrosis or mild/moderate salpingitis isthmica nodosa; severe limitation in mobility
	Nonfunctional	Complete tubal obstruction, extensive fibrosis or salpingitis isthmica nodosa
Fimbria	Mild	Slight injury to fimbria with minimal scarring
	Moderate	Moderate injury to fimbria, with moderate scarring, moderate loss of fimbrial architecture and minimal intrafimbrial fibrosis
	Severe	Severe injury to fimbria, with severe scarring, severe loss of fimbrial architecture and moderate intrafimbrial fibrosis
	Nonfunctional	Severe injury to fimbria, with extensive scarring, complete loss of fimbrial architecture, complete tubal occlusion or hydrosalpinx
Ovary	Mild	Normal or almost normal ovarian size; minimal or mild injury to ovarian serosa
	Moderate	Ovarian size reduced by one-third or more; moderate injury to ovarian surface
	Severe	Ovarian size reduced by two-thirds or more; severe injury to ovarian surface
	Nonfunctional	Ovary absent or completely encased in adhesions

Newer Thoughts on Etiopathology, Staging, and Guidelines

TABLE 3: Endometriosis fertility index classification.[16]

Historical factors			Surgical factors		
Factor	Description	Points	Factor	Description	Points
Age			LF score		
	If age is ≤35 years	2		If LF score = 7–8 (high score)	3
	If age is 36–39 years	1		If LF score = 4–6 (moderate score)	2
	If age is ≥40 years	0		If LF score = 1–3 (low score)	0
Years infertile			AFS endometriosis score		
	If years infertile is ≤3	2		If AFS endometriosis lesion score is < 16	1
	If years infertile is > 3	0		If AFS endometriosis lesion score is ≥ 16	0
Prior pregnancy			AFS total score		
	If there is a history of a prior pregnancy	1		If AFS total score is < 71	1
	If there is no history of prior pregnancy	0		If AFS total score is ≥ 71	0
Total historical factors			**Total surgical factors**		

EFI = Total historical factors + Total surgical factors

☐ Historical + ☐ Surgical = ☐ EFI score

TABLE 4: Least function (LF) score at conclusion of surgery.[16]

Score		Description		Left	Right
4	=	Normal	Fallopian tube	☐	☐
3	=	Mild dysfunction			
2	=	Moderate dysfunction	Fimbria	☐	☐
1	=	Severe dysfunction			
0	=	Absent or nonfunctional	Ovary	☐	☐

To calculate the LF score, add together the lowest score for the left side and the lowest score for the right side. If an ovary is absent on one side, the score is obtained by doubling the lowest score on the side with the ovary.

Lowest Score ☐ + ☐ = ☐
Left   Right   **LF score**

FI = bowel disease cranial to the rectosigmoid junction and FO (other) = other locations, such as abdominal wall endometriosis].

The new #Enzian classification focuses on the classification of superficial, ovarian, deep, and extragenital endometriosis, and pelvic adhesions. The #Enzian classification is based on the known Enzian classification for deep endometriosis using three compartments including far locations as described above. In addition, it covers peritoneal involvement (P), ovary (O), intestines (sigmoid colon, small bowel; FI); adhesions, involving the tuboovarian complex (T) and tubal patency. Individual compartments or organ involvement are identified with the initial capital letters, respectively, [P (peritoneum), O (ovary), T (tubo-ovarian unit), A (RVS, vaginal), B (uterosacral), C (rectum, sigmoid colon), F (far)] and are arranged in this order. **(Fig. 1)** The extent of disease is represented by the numbers 1, 2, and 3 in each of the compartments. The severity of disease in paired organs (such as ovaries, tubes,

Newer Thoughts on Etiopathology, Staging, and Guidelines

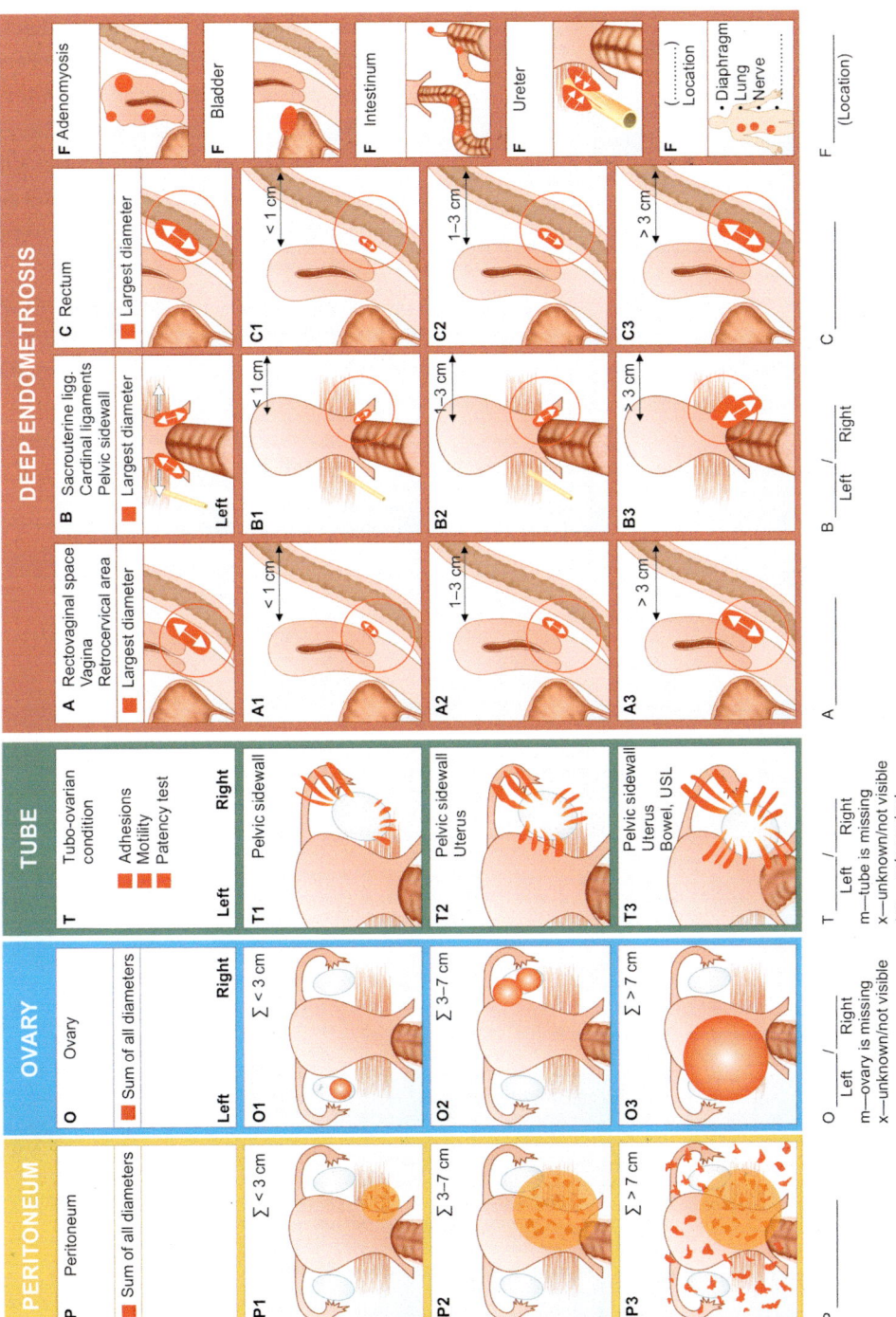

Fig. 1: The #Enzian classification of endometriosis.

uterosacral ligaments, parametrium, ureters) is denoted separately as left/right. Missing or invisible ovary or tube are described with respective suffix (m, missing; x, unknown).[18]

The #Enzian classification has an added advantage to previous listed classifications as location and extent of disease and involvement of retroperitoneal structures including deep infiltrating disease can be described with precision and this classification can be used as a supplement to the rASRM score. This can also provide a relative idea about anticipated operating time. The main disadvantage is the lack of international acceptance. Although the use has been simplified, but still rASRM has a better score in regard to user compatibility.

AAGL Classification

Mauricio S Abrao et al. conducted a multicenter study which included a total of 1,224 patients all of whom were undergoing surgery for endometriosis. The main objective of the study was to decipher a classification which could give a better insight into surgical complexity in relation to patient symptomatology. The AAGL classification gave scores based upon the extent of the disease and finally staging was done from I to IV depending upon the score **(Fig. 2)**. The said classification was compared with ASRM staging system and it was concluded that the former classification allowed for better

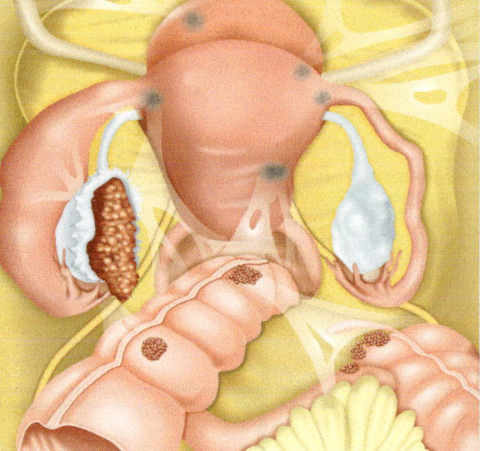

Superficial	Score
<3 cm	2
≥3 cm	4
Vagina (muscularis)	**Score**
<3 cm	5
≥3 cm	8
Left ovary	**Score**
Superficial	2
<3 cm	5
≥3 cm	7
Left ureter	**Score**
Extrinsic	6
Intrinsic	8
Hydroureter	9
Left fallopian tube	**Score**
Slight serosal involvement/damage	2
Moderate immobility	4
Severe immobility	6
Complete obstruction	7
Cul-de-sac obliteration	**Score**
Partial	6
Complete	9
Rectum/Sigmoid colon	**Score**
<3 cm	7
≥3 cm	9
Rectovaginal septum	**Score**
Present	8

Retrocervical	Score
<3 cm	5
≥3 cm	8
Bladder detrusor	**Score**
<3 cm	5
≥3 cm	7
Right ovary	**Score**
Superficial	2
<3 cm	5
≥3 cm	7
Right ureter	**Score**
Extrinsic	6
Intrinsic	8
Hydroureter	9
Right fallopian tube	**Score**
Slight serosal involvement/damage	2
Moderate immobility	4
Severe immobility	6
Complete obstruction	7
Small bowel cecum	**Score**
<3 cm	6
≥3 cm	8
Appendix	**Score**
Present	5

AAGL endometriosis stage	Total score
Stage 1	≤8
Stage 2	9–15
Stage 3	16–15
Stage 4	>21

Fig. 2: The American Association of Gynecologic Laparoscopists (AAGL) classification on endometriosis.[19]

discrimination in intraoperative surgical complexity.[19]

The AAGL 2021 Endometriosis Classification score has the potential to improve clarity in communication within medical records and in clinical research.

■ CONCLUSION

There have been almost 22 published classifications on endometriosis between 1973 and 2021. There is still no international consensus on which specific classification to be used. Classifications have been evolving over the years depending upon the parameters which are studied ranging from symptomatology to its impact on quality of life and infertility to the extent of disease and surgical complexity. To summarize, the #ENZIAN classification system holds its importance for surgical description of deep infiltrating endometriosis. Likewise, EFI classification focused on extent of disease and its impact on fertility. Likewise, the AAGL classification focuses on intraoperative complexity. sASRM scoring still holds importance for the basics that have been taken into account and the ease with which it can be comprehended which improves the communication between the gynecologist and the patient.

■ REFERENCES

1. World Health Organization (WHO). International Classification of Diseases, 11th Revision (ICD-11). Geneva: WHO; 2018.
2. Kennedy S, Bergqvist A, Chapron C, D'Hooghe T, Dunselman G, Greb R, et al. ESHRE guideline for the diagnosis and treatment of endometriosis. Hum Reprod. 2005;20:2698-2704.
3. International working group of AAGL ESGE ESHRE and WES, Johnson N, Petrozza J, Tomassetti C, Abrao MS, Einarsson JI, AWH, Lee TTM, Missmer S, Vermeulen N, et al. An International Glossary on Endometriosis (submitted for publication) 2021
4. Dunselman GAJ, Vermeulen N, Becker C, Calhaz-Jorge C, D'Hooghe T, De Bie B, et al. ESHRE guideline: management of women with endometriosis. Hum Reprod. 2014;29(3):400-12.
5. Sourial S, Tempest N, Hapangama DK. Theories on the pathogenesis of endometriosis. Int J Reprod Med. 2014;2014: 179515.
6. Uğur M, Turan C, Mungan T, Kuşçu E, Senöz S, Ağiş HT, et al. Endometriosis in association with müllerian anomalies. Gynecol Obstet Invest. 1995;40(4):261-4.
7. Marsh EE, Laufer MR. Endometriosis in premenarcheal girls who do not have an associated obstructive anomaly. Fertil Steril. 2005;83(3):758-60.
8. Channabasavaiah AD, Joseph JV. Thoracic endometriosis: revisiting the association between clinical presentation and thoracic pathology based on thoracoscopic findings in 110 patients. Medicine (Baltimore). 2010; 89:183.
9. Ferguson BR, Bennington JL, Haber SL. Histochemistry of mucosubstances and histology of mixed mullerian pelvic lymph node glandular inclusions. Evidence for histogenesis by mullerian metaplasia of coelomic epithelium. Obstet Gynecol. 1969; 33(5):617-25.
10. Rahmioglu N, Nyholt DR, Morris AP, Missmer SA, Montgomery GW, Zondervan KT. Genetic variants underlying risk of endometriosis: insights from meta-analysis of eight genome-wide association and replication datasets. Hum Reprod Update. 2014;20:702-16.
11. Anglesio MS, Papadopoulos N, Ayhan A, Nazeran TM, Noë M, Horlings HM, et al. Cancer-associated mutations in endometriosis without cancer. N Engl J Med. 2017; 376:1835.
12. Bulun SE, Wan Y, Matei D. Epithelial Mutations in Endometriosis: Link to Ovarian Cancer. Endocrinology. 2019;160:626.
13. De Cicco C, Corona R, Schonman R, et al. Bowel resection for deep endometriosis: a systematic review. BJOG 2011; 118:285.

14. Brosens IA, Puttemans PJ, Deprest J. The endoscopic localization of endometrial implants in the ovarian chocolate cyst. Fertil Steril. 1994;61:1034.
15. Revised American Society for Reproductive Medicine classification of endometriosis: 1996. Fertil Steril. 1997;67:817-21.
16. Adamson GD, Pasta DJ. Endometriosis fertility index: the new, validated endometriosis staging system. Fertil Steril. 2010;94(5):1609-15.
17. Tuttlies F, Keckstein J, Ulrich U, Possover M, Schweppe KW, Wustlich M, et al. ENZIAN-score, a classification of deep infiltrating endometriosis. Zentralbl Gynakol. 2005; 127:275-81.
18. Keckstein J, Saridogan E, Ulrich UA, Sillem M, Oppelt P, Schweppe KW, et al. The #Enzian classification: A comprehensive non-invasive and surgical description system for endometriosis. Acta Obstet Gynecol Scand. 2021;1001165-75.
19. Abrao MS, Andres MP, Miller CE, Gingold JA, Rius M, Neto JS, et al. AAGL 2021 endometriosis classification: An anatomy-based surgical complexity score. J Minim Invasive Gynecol. 2021;28(11):1941-50.e1.

CHAPTER 3

Clinical Presentation: Endometriosis

Kalyan B Barmade, Manisha K Barmade

■ INTRODUCTION

Endometriosis is the presence of endometrial glands and stroma-like lesions outside of the uterus. The lesions present in different parts like peritoneal lesions such as superficial and deep implants or endometrioma ovary or deep infiltrating endometriosis (DIE).[1]

Clinical presentation is variable in various age groups, peak of the disease at 25 and 29 years age group, and lowest in 44 years age group. Patients often presents with intermenstrual bleeding, dysmenorrhea, dyspareunia, dyschezia, and painful urination (dysuria). The pain is usually characterized as chronic, cyclic, and may be sometime progressive in nature.

Women suffering from endometriosis may have experience of hyperalgesia, a phenomenon that indicates neuropathic pain. In DIE, the neural damage is caused by the invasion of endometrial stromal cells and mediators such as serotonin, histamine, prostaglandins, and nerve growth factor. These agents are released from mast cells, activated macrophages, and leukocytes, damages directly the sensory nerve fibers and also present in the peritoneal fluid. There are three subtypes of endometriosis: (1) Superficial peritoneal lesions, (2) the ovarian endometrioma, and (3) DIE. The degree of clinical manifestations of the patient is not directly associated with the extent of the disease or the size of endometriosis lesions.[2]

Endometriotic lesions on ovaries are described as ovarian endometriomas or as pseudocysts, which account for 17–44% in women with endometriosis; these may be bilateral in 50% of the cases, and are twice more frequent in the left ovary. They differentiate from the common ovarian cysts as it is lined by endometrial stroma, epithelium, and glands. Chocolate fluid accumulates, covering the wall and filling in the cyst, containing old, degenerated blood products, like hemosiderin-filled macrophages, pigmented histiocytes resulting in a chocolate-like appearance. DIE refers to endometriotic lesions that infiltrate the peritoneum >5 mm and involve additionally the bladder, the ureter, and the bowel, more frequently the rectovaginal septum, and less commonly the sigmoid. Superficial peritoneal lesions are asymptomatic, they sporadically can cause a thickening or hemorrhage of the mucosa or even be the reason for a pathological cervicovaginal smear. The histologic diagnosis of endometriosis may not show always appearance of the endometrial glands or even the stroma caused by inflammation, edema, or hemorrhage.[2]

Adolescent patients report severe primary dysmenorrhea, which is often resistant to nonsteroidal anti-inflammatory drugs and oral contraceptives. The appearance of peritoneal lesions is also different. In adolescents, endometriotic implants are florid (clear or red papules, vesicular implants) with minimal fibrosis that may lead to obstructive genital tract anomalies, contrast seen in adult patients, and black implants with dense fibrotic tissue. Rectal and bladder endometriosis and uterine adenomyosis are concomitant pathologies.[2] These can be asymptomatic, only coming to a clinician's attention during evaluation for infertility.

Classification of endometriosis-associated pain symptoms have been established by the American Society for Reproductive Medicine (ASRM) based on the morphology of peritoneal and pelvic implants such as red, white, and black lesions; percentage of involvement of each lesion should be included. Number, size, and location endometrial implants, plaques, endometriomas and adhesions should be noted. Endometriosis in bowel, urinary tract, fallopian tube, vagina, cervix, skin, or other locations should be documented per ASRM guidelines. Stages of endometriosis according to ASRM guidelines are stage I, II, III, and IV determined based on the point scores and correspond to minimal, mild, moderate, and severe endometriosis.[1] There are recently many more classifications systems coming up, which indirectly inform about modality of treatment and fertility outcome collaboration.

REFERENCES

1. Parasar P, Ozcan P, Terry KL. Endometriosis: epidemiology, diagnosis and clinical management. Curr Obstet Gynecol Rep. 2017;6(1):34-41. doi: 10.1007/s13669-017-0187-1.
2. Gałczyński K, Jóźwik M, Lewkowicz D, Semczuk-Sikora A, Semczuk A. Ovarian endometrioma: a possible finding in adolescent girls and young women: a mini-review. J Ovarian Res. 2019;12(1):104. doi: 10.1186/s13048-019-0582-5.

CHAPTER 4

Diagnosis of Endometriosis

Aruna Suman, Panchampreet Kaur

INTRODUCTION

Endometriosis is defined as a disease characterized by the presence of endometrium-like epithelium and/or stroma outside the endometrium and myometrium, usually with an associated inflammatory process.[1] It causes scarring and fibrosis. The growth of endometriotic tissue is mostly found in reproductive age group. However, the clinical consequences can have long-term effect on a woman's physical, sexual, psychological, and social life.[2] The diagnosis of endometriosis involves high degree of clinical suspicion and this can be further supported by testing which includes markers, imaging studies and endoscopy. The framework for diagnosis is enumerated as under and is discussed in detail.

- General testing
- Markers
- Imaging
- Contrast imaging
- Laparoscopy

Diagnosis is established on the basis of history and clinical evaluation complemented by imaging, surgery alone, or in combination. A woman is advised to keep a symptom diary so as to aid diagnosis and further management. Endometriosis should especially be suspected in the presence of a triad of symptoms of subfertility, dysmenorrhea, dyspareunia. Extragenital endometriosis may be asymptomatic even in advanced disease in ovarian or rectovaginal endometriosis or may present with hematuria when bladder is involved. The menstrual disturbances might include short cycles, heavy menstruation, and longer flow duration.

Examination should comprise a complete general and systemic examination. Per abdomen examination should be done after ensuring empty bladder. Bimanual examination may reveal adnexal masses and pelvic signs such as restricted mobility with or without tender nodularity in the posterior fornix. Always a combined per vaginum and rectal examination should be done to rule out pouch of Douglas (POD) nodularity. Occasionally, endometriotic lesions are seen during per speculum examination. It has also been seen and reported that examination during menstruation increases the probability of specific diagnosis of endometriosis. Severe, persistent, and recurrent symptoms with pelvic signs or deep endometriosis may involve the bowel, bladder, ureter, or extra-pelvic endometriosis.

There have been numerous studies on the role of biomarkers in the establishment of diagnosis of endometriosis but further research is warranted.[3] Recently, guidelines by ESHRE (European Society of Human Reproduction and Embryology) have stated that measurement of biomarkers in endometrial tissue, blood, menstrual or uterine fluids should not be used by clinicians to diagnose endometriosis.[4] We would be discussing in brief about the various biomarkers available to provide a broader perspective because this might hold the future of endometriosis diagnosis.

■ BLOOD BIOMARKERS

Various biomarkers available for testing are mostly glycoproteins, growth factors, or proteins related to immunology or angiogenesis or hormones.[5]

- *Glycoproteins:*
  - *Cancer antigen 125 (CA 125):* Its role either alone or in combination with other markers such as type 1 mRNA, and monocyte chemoattractant protein-1 (MCP-1) has been studied.[6,7] It is a non-specific marker of inflammation. Normal values are below 35 U/mL. Very high values are indicative of ovarian cancer. However, levels might be abnormal in endometriosis, tuberculosis, pelvic inflammatory disease, fibroids, liver disease, and even pregnancy.
  - *CA 19-9:* Few studies have reported the association between CA 19-9 and endometriosis.[6] However, it has also been seen to have lower sensitivity as compared to CA 125 for the detection of endometriosis.[8]
  - *Follistatin:* It is an inhibitor of activin.[9] It has been reported to be specifically increased in ovarian endometriosis and thereby distinguish from other benign cysts. More studies are needed to validate its further importance.[10]
  - *Glycodelin A:* It is a 28 kDa glycoprotein. It has been reported to be seen in increased concentrations in serum and peritoneal fluid in women with ovarian endometriosis and thereby can be used in adjunct with other biomarkers for diagnosis of endometriosis.[11]
- *Immunological markers and inflammatory cytokines:* Interleukin 1 (IL-1), IL-6, IL-8, tumor necrosis factor alpha, MCP-1, and interferon gamma (IFN-γ) have been studied.[6] The inflammatory marker C-reactive protein (CRP) has been seen to be associated but again it is a nonspecific marker of inflammatory process.
- Soluble intercellular molecule-1 (sICAM-1) levels have been reported to increase during early stages of endometriosis (I–II) and decrease at stage III–IV. The elevation of cell adhesion molecule osteopontin and matrix metalloproteinases (MMPs) has also been documented.[5]
- *Angiogenesis:* Vascular endothelial growth factor (VEGF), pigment epithelium-derived factor (PEDF), soluble epidermal growth factor (EGF), and platelet-derived growth factor (PDGF), hepatocyte growth factor (HGF), fibroblast growth factor-2 (FGF-2), angiogenin, and soluble Flt-1 (VEGFR-1) in serum of women with endometriosis have been studied but their role has been inconclusive.[5]
- *Autoantibodies:* Total immunoglobulin levels and antiendometrial antibodies have been investigated as biomarkers for endometriosis.[6] In patients with ovarian endometrioma autoantibodies against insulin-like growth factor 2 and mRNA-binding protein 1 (IMP1) have been found to be significant.[5]
- *Micro RNAs (miRNAs):* miRNAs are short, noncoding sequences that regulate gene expression at the posttranscriptional level.[5] They may be released into the circulation and are protected from endogenous RNase degradation because of inclusion within exosomes or association with specific protein complexes. These are emerging as potential molecular indicators to noninvasively identify endometriosis.[12]

- *Proteomics:* A variety of studies have been published regarding protein "fingerprints" for the diagnosis of endometriosis; however, proteomics technologies are costly and time-consuming.[5,13,14]

URINE BIOMARKERS

Urine-based biomarkers have been reported to be used individually or in combination with other panel of markers. Various markers that have been studied include Creatinine-corrected soluble fms-like tyrosine kinase-1 (sFlt-1), cytokeratin-19 (CK19), and MMPs.[15-17]

ENDOMETRIAL BIOMARKERS

The endometrial biomarkers are more invasive than serology. The endometrial tissue is retrieved through an endometrial aspiration biopsy done in office setting. It should be done in the proliferative phase in order to avoid affecting an inadvertent pregnancy. These biomarkers involve endometrial transcriptome, miRNAs, and neuronal markers. These form a part of research studies.[5]

A recent Cochrane review update had also stated that no reliable biomarkers are available for clinical use currently. They should at present be undertaken only in a research setting.[18,19]

IMAGING STUDIES

Ultrasound

Transvaginal scan (TVS) is a good tool to diagnose ovarian endometriosis masses larger than 10 mm. The characteristic feature is the presence of diffuse low level internal echoes and hyperechoic foci in the walls (classic chocolate cyst). TVS helps in determining the type of mass, cystic, mixed or solid mass, and the shape and location also can be identified. The classic sonographic appearance of endometrioma is homogeneous hypoechoic lesion with low or medium level echoes and no internal vascularity, referred to as ground-glass appearance **(Figs. 1A and B)**.

Endometrial stromal tissue may show presence of Doppler-detected blood flow. Chronic endometrioma may mimic solid masses due to presence of older blood products and fibrosis. Endometriotic cyst might be confused with hemorrhagic cyst. However, hemorrhagic cyst resolves after some days while endometrioma does not.

Magnetic Resonance Imaging

Magnetic resonance imaging (MRI) can be a helpful diagnostic modality whenever in doubt. It shows characteristic finding of increased signal intensity on T1-weighted

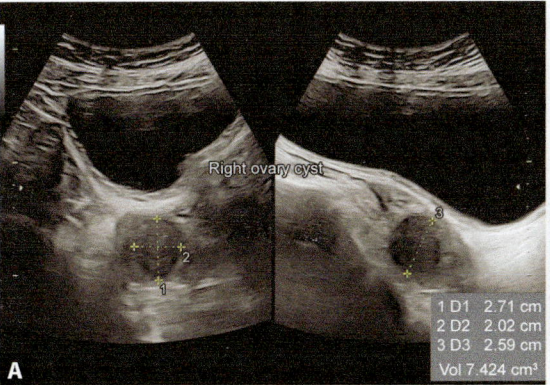
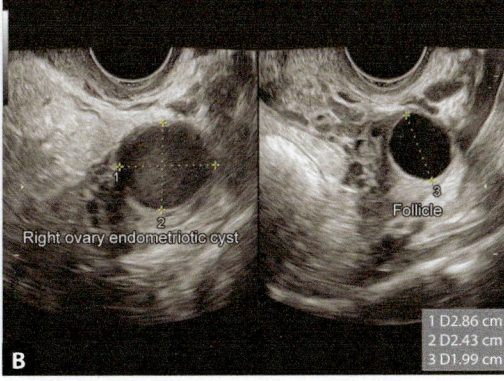

Figs. 1A and B: Transabdominal (A) and transvaginal (B) images showing an endometriotic cyst.

images and decreased signal intensity on T2-weighted images. MRI is a noninvasive, nonionizing radiation, which consistently demonstrates anatomic tissue planes and is more valuable than computed tomography (CT). It can detect hemorrhagic nature of masses too. MRI cannot be used to detect extraovarian endometrial adhesions and intraperitoneal implants, nor can it correlate with surgical assessment of severity.

Computed Tomography Scan

Computed tomography scan gathers anatomical information from cross-sectional planes but is rarely used as a diagnostic method owing to differing appearances of lesions. Differential diagnosis of endometriosis and peritoneal carcinomatosis can be difficult.

Clinicians are recommended to use imaging [ultrasound (US) or MRI] in the diagnostic workup for endometriosis, but they need to be aware that a negative finding does not exclude endometriosis, particularly superficial peritoneal disease.[4] The endometriotic implants in anterior abdominal wall can be demonstrated on sonography using a high-resolution linear transducer. The classic findings are solid, heterogeneous, hypoechoic mass with scattered internal echoes, with sometimes areas of cystic change with spiculated margins, with some vascularity on Doppler evaluation. The endometriotic cyst rupture is a surgical emergency and would appear as complex free fluid compatible with hemoperitoneum in addition to a hemorrhagic-appearing adnexal mass.

■ LAPAROSCOPY (FIGS. 2A AND B)

The diagnosis of endometriosis is confirmatory when lesions are directly visualized during surgical approach along with histologic confirmation of endometrial glands and stroma in biopsies of suspected lesions. However, there are risks involving surgical complications. Laparoscopy was considered the gold standard for diagnosing endometriosis. However, recent guidelines by ESHRE have stated that laparoscopy is no longer the diagnostic gold standard and it is now only recommended in patients with negative imaging results and/or where empirical treatment was unsuccessful or inappropriate.[4] A skilled advanced laparoscopic surgeon should be involved. During laparoscopy, pelvis can be obscured by adhesions masking the findings making the approach difficult. Currently, pelvic/abdominal disease is clinically subdivided into superficial (peritoneal/serosal) lesions,

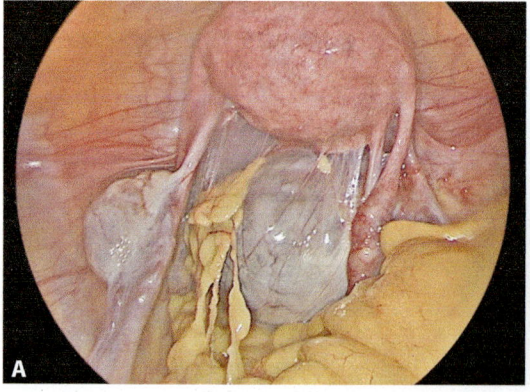
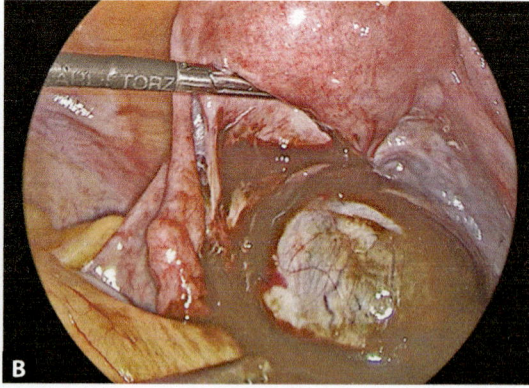

Figs. 2A and B: Laparoscopic images show (A) pelvic adhesions and (B) chocolate-colored fluid draining from endometriotic cyst.

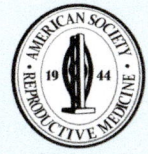

	Endometriosis	<1 cm	1–3 cm	>3 cm
Peritoneum	Superficial	1	2	4
	Deep	2	4	6
Ovary	R Superficial	1	2	4
	Deep	4	16	20
	L Superficial	1	2	4
	Deep	4	16	20
	Posterior cul-de-sac obliteration	Partial		Complete
		4		40
	Adhesions	<1/3 enclosure	1/3–2/3 enclosure	>2/3 enclosure
Ovary	R Filmy	1	2	4
	Dense	4	8	16
	L Filmy	1	2	4
	Dense	4	8	16
Tube	R Filmy	1	2	4
	Dense	4*	8*	16
	L Filmy	1	2	4
	Dense	4*	8*	16

Patient's name_____ Date_____
Stage I (Minimal) — 1–5   Laparoscopy_____Laparotomy_____Photography_____
Stage II (Mild) — 6–15   Recommended treatment_____
Stage III (Moderate) — 16–40
Stage IV (Severe) — >40
Total_____   Prognosis_____

*If the fimbriated end of the fallopian tube is completely enclosed, change the point assignment to 16.
Denote appearance of superficial implant types as red [(R), red, red-pink, flamelike, vesicular blobs, clear vesicles], white [(W), opacifications, peritoneal defects, yellow-brown], or black [(B), black, hemosiderin deposits, blue]. Denote percent of total described as R___%, W___% and B___%. Total should equal 100%.

Fig. 3: American Society for Reproductive Medicine (ASRM) revised classification of endometriosis.

ovarian endometriosis cysts (endometrioma), and deep endometriosis (by arbitrary definition >5 mm below the serosal/peritoneal surface).[20] Biopsy from the site can be considered at the time of diagnostic laparoscopy, but a negative histological test does not rule out its presence. Red lesions are seen more frequently than burnt lesions. If a lesion is not visible on laparoscopy, biopsy from POD should be taken and sent for histopathology. Both diagnostic laparoscopy and imaging combined with empirical treatment (hormonal contraceptives or progestogens) can be considered in women suspected of endometriosis. There is no evidence of superiority of either approach and pros and cons should be discussed with the patient.[4] **Figure 3** shows the endometriosis classification as per American Society for Reproductive Medicine (ASRM).[21]

CONCLUSION

The diagnosis of endometriosis involves good clinical acumen and a detailed history along with examination usually helps clinch the diagnosis. Newer biomarkers are available but these are still an area of research to actually incorporate them into clinical practice. Ultrasound can supplement the clinical diagnosis. An advanced pelvic laparoscopic surgeon should be involved and endoscopy is recommended in symptomatic patients with negative imaging studies and/or where empirical treatment has been unsuccessful or not indicated.

REFERENCES

1. International working group of AAGL ESGE ESHRE and WES; Johnson N, Petrozza J, Tomassetti C, Abrao MS, Einarsson JI, AW H, et al. An International Glossary on Endometriosis (submitted for publication). 2021.
2. Culley L, Law C, Hudson N, Denny E, Mitchell H, Baumgarten M, et al. The social and psychological impact of endometriosis on women's lives: a critical narrative review. Hum Reprod Update. 2013;19:625-39.
3. Anastasiu CV, Moga MA, Elena Neculau A, Bălan A, Scârneciu I, Dragomir RM, et al. Biomarkers for the Noninvasive Diagnosis of Endometriosis: State of the Art and Future Perspectives. Int J Mol Sci. 2020;21(5):1750.
4. European Society of Human Reproduction and Embryology. (2022). ESHRE Guideline Endometriosis. [online] Available from https://www.eshre.eu/-/media/sitecore-files/Guidelines/Endometriosis/ESHRE-GUIDELINE-ENDOMETRIOSIS-2022_2.pdf [Last accessed September, 2023].
5. Fassbender A, Burney RO, O DF, D'Hooghe T, Giudice L. Update on Biomarkers for the Detection of Endometriosis. Biomed Res Int. 2015;2015:130854.
6. May KE, Conduit-Hulbert SA, Villar J, Kirtley S, Kennedy SH, Becker CM. Peripheral biomarkers of endometriosis: a systematic review. Hum Reprod Update. 2010;16(6): 651-74.
7. Agic A, Djalali S, Wolfler MM, Halis G, Diedrich K, Hornung D. Combination of CCR1 mRNA, MCP1, and CA125 measurements in peripheral blood as a diagnostic test for endometriosis. Reprod Sci. 2008;15(9):906-11.
8. Harada T, Kubota T, Aso T. Usefulness of CA19-9 versus CA125 for the diagnosis of endometriosis. Fertil Steril. 2002;78:733-9.
9. de Winter JP, ten Dijke P, de Vries CJ, van Achterberg TA, Sugino H, de Waele P, et al. Follistatins neutralize activin bioactivity by inhibition of activin binding to its type II receptors. Mol Cell Endocrinol. 1996;116: 105-14.
10. Florio P, Reis FM, Torres PB, Calonaci F, Abrao MS, Nascimento LL, et al. High serum follistatin levels in women with ovarian endometriosis. Hum Reprod. 2009;24(10): 2600-6.
11. Kocbek V, Vouk K, Mueller MD, Rižner TL, Bersinger NA. Elevated glycodelin-A concentrations in serum and peritoneal fluid of women with ovarian endometriosis. Gynecol Endocrinol. 2013;29(5):455-9.
12. Bjorkman S, Taylor HS. MicroRNAs in endometriosis: biological function and emerging biomarker candidates. Biol Reprod. 2019;100(5):1135-46.
13. Fassbender A, Waelkens E, Verbeeck N, Kyama CM, Bokor A, Vodolazkaia A, et al. Proteomics analysis of plasma for early diagnosis of endometriosis. Obstet Gynecol. 2012;119(2 Pt 1):276-85.
14. Zheng N, Pan C, Liu W. New serum biomarkers for detection of endometriosis using matrix-assisted laser desorption/ionization time-of-flight mass spectrometry. J Int Med Res. 2011;39(4):1184-92.
15. Cho SH, Oh YJ, Nam A, Kim HY, Park JH, Kim JH, et al. Evaluation of serum and urinary angiogenic factors in patients with endometriosis. Am J Reprod Immunol. 2007; 58(6):497-504.
16. Tokushige N, Markham R, Crossett B, Ahn SB, Nelaturi VL, Khan A, et al. Discovery of a novel biomarker in the urine in women

with endometriosis. Fertil Steril. 2011;95(1): 46-9.
17. Becker CM, Louis G, Exarhopoulos A, Mechsner S, Ebert AD, Zurakowski D, et al. Matrix metalloproteinases are elevated in the urine of patients with endometriosis. Fertil Steril. 2010;94(6):2343-6.
18. Gupta D, Hull ML, Fraser I, Miller L, Bossuyt PM, Johnson N, et al. Endometrial biomarkers for the non-invasive diagnosis of endometriosis. Cochrane Database Syst Rev. 2016;4(4):CD012165.
19. Nisenblat V, Bossuyt PM, Shaikh R, Farquhar C, Jordan V, Scheffers CS, et al. Blood biomarkers for the non-invasive diagnosis of endometriosis. Cochrane Database Syst Rev. 2016;2016(5):CD012179.
20. Cornillie FJ, Oosterlynck D, Lauweryns JM, Koninckx PR. Deeply infiltrating pelvic endometriosis: histology and clinical significance. Fertil Steril. 1990;53:978-83.
21. Revised American Society for Reproductive Medicine classification of endometriosis: 1996. Fertil Steril. 1997;67(5):817-21.

CHAPTER 5

Endometriosis Scoring Systems

Monisha Singh, Narendra Malhotra, Neharika Malhotra, Jaideep Malhotra

■ INTRODUCTION

Endometriosis is a debilitating disease and difficult to diagnose for proper management strategies, and good scoring systems are needed. This chapter discusses the scoring and classification of the disease and its clinical relevance.

■ DEFINITION

Endometriosis is a chronic gynecologic disease characterized by the development and presence of histological elements such as endometrial glands and stroma in anatomical positions and organs outside of the uterine cavity. There are several developed theories about the etiology of endometriosis based on the logical sequel relating the severity of symptoms to the stage of the disease, although none of these proposed models can fully explain the range of clinical manifestations of the disease.

The diagnosis of endometriosis in the majority of women is often delayed, and thus women unavoidably suffer from the pain and the long-term effects of this debilitating disease, including infertility. In women with infertility, endometriosis has been found to be up to 50%, whereas in adolescents, the incidence of endometriosis is reported to be 47% of those who have experienced laparoscopy for pelvic pain.[1]

Classification (Fig. 1)

According to the International Working Group of the American Association of Gynecologic Laparoscopists (AAGL), European Society of Gynecologic Endoscopy (ESGE), European Society of Human Reproduction and Embryology (ESHRE), and World Endometriosis Society (WES), *superficial endometriosis* is defined by the presence of endometrium-like tissue involving the peritoneal surface. The lesions can have different appearances and colors, e.g., clear and black.[2] In contrast, the same group defines *deep endometriosis* (DE) as endometrium-like tissue lesions in the abdomen that extend on or under the peritoneal surface. They are usually nodular, able to invade adjacent structures, and associated with fibrosis and the disruption of normal anatomy.[2] *Ovarian endometriosis* is defined as endometrium-like tissue in the form of ovarian cysts.[2] Endometriomas may be either invagination cysts or true cysts, with the cyst wall also containing endometrial-like tissue and dark blood-stained fluid.

The ovary is a common site affected by endometriosis.[3] The intrapelvic localizations of endometriosis include involvement of the uterosacral ligaments (USLs), vagina, rectum, rectovaginal space, or bladder (frequently at the posterior bladder dome).[4] Endometriosis

Endometriosis Scoring Systems

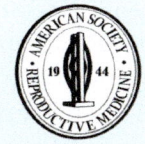

American Society for Reproductive Medicine
Revised Classification of Endometriosis

Patient's name_____ Date_____

Stage I   (Minimal)   — 1–5   Laparoscopy_____ Laparotomy_____ Photography_____
Stage II   (Mild)   — 6–15   Recommended treatment_____
Stage III (Moderate)   — 16–40
Stage IV   (Severe)   — >40
Total_____   Prognosis_____

	Endometriosis	<1 cm	1–3 cm	>3 cm
Peritoneum	Superficial	1	2	4
	Deep	2	4	6
Ovary	R Superficial	1	2	4
	Deep	4	16	20
	L Superficial	1	2	4
	Deep	4	16	20
	Posterior cul-de-sac obliteration	Partial		Complete
		4		40
	Adhesions	<1/3 enclosure	1/3–2/3 enclosure	>2/3 enclosure
Ovary	R Filmy	1	2	4
	Dense	4	8	16
	L Filmy	1	2	4
	Dense	4	8	16
Tube	R Filmy	1	2	4
	Dense	4*	8*	16
	L Filmy	1	2	4
	Dense	4*	8*	16

*If the fimbriated end of the fallopian tube is completely enclosed, change the point assignment to 16.
Denote appearance of superficial implant types as red [(R), red, red-pink, flamelike, vesicular blobs, clear vesicles], white [(W), opacifications, peritoneal defects, yellow-brown], or black [(B), black, hemosiderin deposits, blue]. Denote percent of total described as R___%, W___% and B___%. Total should equal 100%.

Additional endometriosis_____   Associated pathology: _____

To be used with normal tubes and ovaries   L   R

To be used with abnormal tubes and/or ovaries   L   R

Fig. 1: The 1996 revised endometriosis classification system based on ASRM classification gave a detailed intraoperative picture of degree of endometriosis.
Source: Adapted from Revised ASRM classification. American Society for Reproductive Medicine (1996).

can also affect extrapelvic organs, such as the abdominal wall, diaphragm, and nerves.

Endometriosis Fertility Index

The purpose of the development of the endometriosis fertility index (EFI) system is to predict the pregnancy rate in patients with surgically documented endometriosis who have not attempted to become pregnant with in vitro fertilization (IVF). Functional scores are determined by the surgeon and range from 0 to 4 points as follows: Absent or nonfunctional as 0, severe dysfunction as 1, moderate dysfunction as 2, mild dysfunction as 3, and normal as 4. Not only the least functional score, but also other surgical factors such as revised American Society for Reproductive Medicine (rASRM) total score and endometriosis lesion score of rASRM are included. Finally, the EFI score is calculated by summing the historical and surgical scores and ranges from 0 to 10 points, with 10 indicating the best prognosis and 0 the worst prognosis.

Enzian Classification

The revised Enzian classification was simplified by dividing retroperitoneal structures into three compartments **(Fig. 2)**.[5] The posterior part of the uterus was divided into compartment A consisting of the rectovaginal septum and vagina, compartment B consisting of the uterosacral ligament and pelvic walls, and compartment C consisting of the sigmoid colon and rectum. The severity of the lesion is set to invasiveness <1 cm for grade 1, invasiveness 1–3 cm for grade 2, and invasiveness >3 cm for grade 3. The prefix "E" indicates the presence of a tumor of endometriosis. The number that follows the prefix indicates the size of the lesion, and after the number, the lowercase English letter indicates the affected compartment. Because of the poor level of international acceptance and complexity with alphanumeric grading, it is not widely recognized, though further study and modification may bring the Enzian score to light.

There are a number of imaging tests that can be used to diagnose endometriosis, including:

- *Transvaginal sonography (TVS):* TVS is the first-line imaging technique in the diagnosis of pelvic endometriosis and in particular for deep infiltrating endometriosis (DIE).[3] It is important to note, however, that there is substantial heterogeneity in the reported sensitivity and specificity of TVS with regard to detection of DIE, irrespective of its location.
- Another technique described by some authors is rectal endoscopic ultrasonography (REU).
- *Magnetic resonance imaging (MRI):* This test uses a strong magnetic field and radio waves to create detailed images of the body. MRI is more sensitive than ultrasound for detecting endometriosis, and it can also be used to see how deep the endometriosis has spread.
- Another imaging technique that can be used for the detection of endometriosis is the *multidetector computerized tomography enema* (MDCT-e). This is an MDCT with colonic distension obtained with water. One of the advantages of MDCT-e is the potential to study the entire bowel with a differential diagnosis from other pathologies, such as cancer or inflammatory disease.
- A different approach is computed tomography colonography (CTC), also named virtual colonoscopy. It can be used to identify only rectosigmoid endometriosis and estimates the degree of intestinal stenosis.

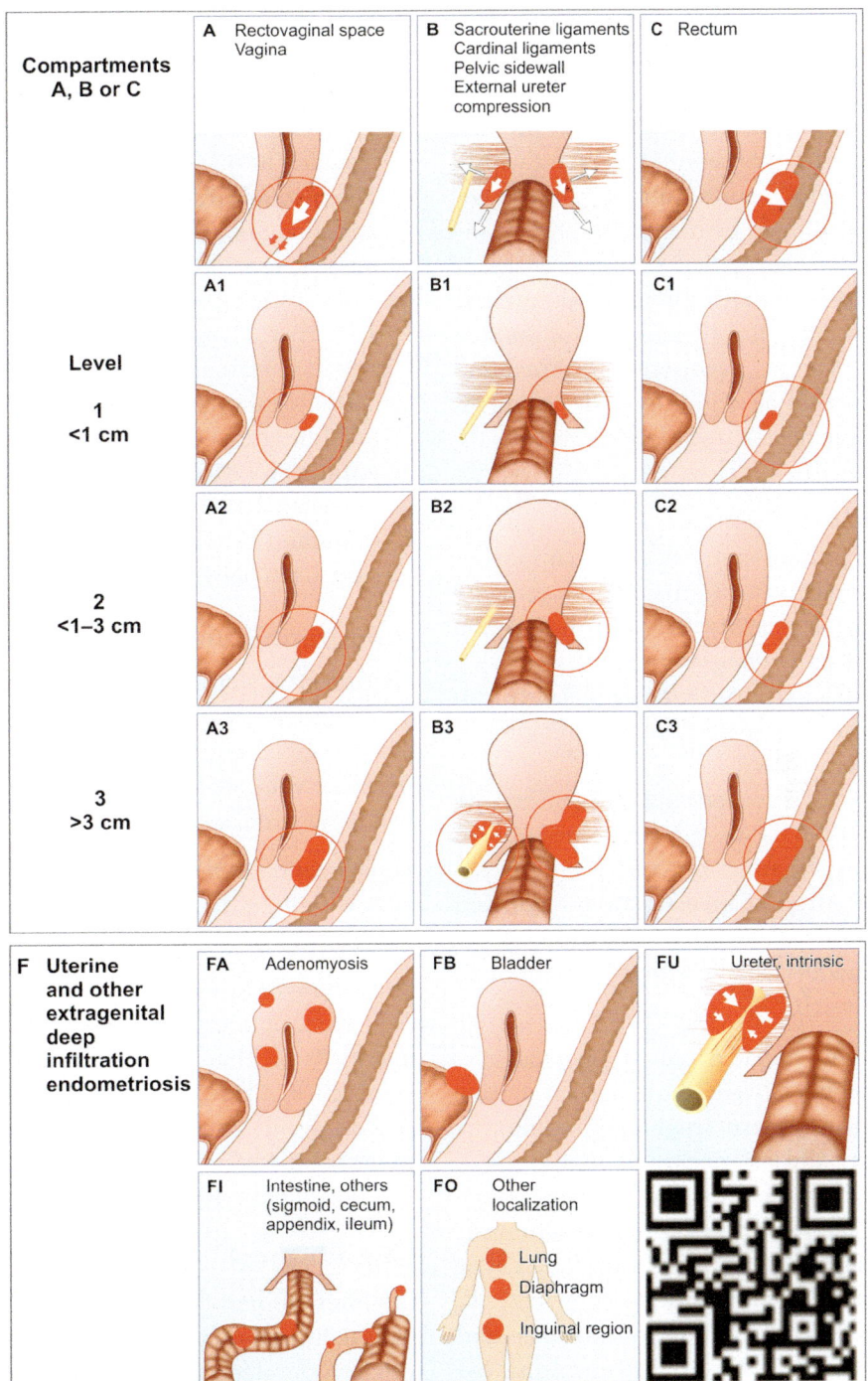

Fig. 2: Enzian classification of deep infiltrating endometriosis [according to the Endometriosis Research Foundation (SEF)].
Source: Keckstein©

- *Laparoscopy:* It is the current gold standard for definitive diagnosis, staging, and treatment. Its greatest benefit is its ability to do maximal cytoreduction at the first surgical intervention. However, for this, an appropriate and trained laparoscopic surgeon should be the one to provide the first surgical expertise. Surgical excision of DIE is risky, requiring long operating times and excellent technical skills. For the very same reasons, preoperative ultrasound mapping of all endometriotic lesions is therefore necessary before surgery.

Reasons to assess endometriosis extent prior to intervention are:
- When to intervene—to go for surgical or nonsurgical intervention
- Fertility specialists can plan appropriate fertility-enhancing surgeries.
- Multidisciplinary team availability can be there at the time of surgery (colorectal involvement).
- To assess whether such a case can be managed at their setup or to be referred to a tertiary laparoscopic center

The method of investigating suspected endometriosis should start alongside rigorous history taking. There is no scope of wait and watch.

The following should be noted specifically:
- Age, height, weight, ethnic origin, parity, bleeding pattern (regular, irregular, or absent), and last menstrual period
- Previous surgery for endometriosis (type and effect) and previous myomectomy or cesarean delivery (these entail increased risk of DIE in the bladder)
- Family history of endometriosis and previous nonsurgical treatment for endometriosis (type, duration, and effect)
- Subfertility including duration of subfertility
- Treatment for infertility and outcome of fertility treatment
- Pain (dysmenorrhea, dyspareunia, dysuria, dyschezia, and chronic pelvic pain)
- Hematochezia and/or hematuria
- The onset and duration of symptoms should be noted and, if possible, the intensity of the pain recorded by letting the patient use a visual analog scale or investigating it with a 0–10 narrative numeric rating scale.
- Pelvic examination should include speculum examination (direct visualization of vaginal or cervical DIE) and vaginal palpation. Mobility, fixation, and/or tenderness of the uterus should be evaluated carefully. Site-specific tenderness in the pelvis should also be evaluated.

Sonographic View

Ovarian endometrioma: The most common appearance is a unilocular cyst with ground glass echogenicity of the cyst fluid. Endometrioma with papillation are more common in older women.

Superficial endometriosis: Ultrasound provides with poor diagnosis of such superficial endometriosis.

Deep endometriosis: With a sonographic view, there is a lack of uniformity while discussing about DIE location and the extent of disease. As of 2016, there was lack of consensus leading to poor description of appearance, poor classification of disease location, and difficulty in pool study.

IDEA Protocol

The International Deep Endometriosis Analysis (IDEA) group is a consortium of experts who have developed a consensus statement on the use of imaging to diagnose endometriosis.[6] The IDEA statement includes a standardized protocol for TVS that can be used to detect and characterize endometriosis. In addition to terms, definitions and measurements to describe the sonographic features of DIE, adhesions, and adenomyosis and endometriomas, this consensus opinion includes recommendations regarding how to take a history, how to perform a clinical examination, how to perform an ultrasound examination, and which ultrasound modality to use when examining patients with suspected or known endometriosis. DIE anatomical locations in this consensus were modified from Chapron's anatomical distribution of pelvic DIE.

The IDEA protocol is a valuable tool for clinicians who are managing women with endometriosis. It is more accurate than standard TVS, provides more information about the extent of disease, and is a standardized approach that can improve communication between clinicians.

The specific steps involved in the IDEA protocol for endometriosis scanning are as follows:
1. The patient is placed in the lithotomy position and a TVS probe is inserted into the vagina.
2. The probe is used to image the pelvis in four planes—sagittal, transverse, right oblique, and left oblique.
3. The examiner looks for the presence of any of the features listed in the IDEA protocol, including ovarian endometriomas, DIE, and adhesions.
4. If any of these features are found, the examiner measures their size and depth.
5. The examiner then interprets the findings of the scan using the standardized system provided by the IDEA protocol.

The IDEA protocol **(Table 1)** consists of:
- *Imaging planes:* The IDEA protocol specifies four imaging planes that should be evaluated during TVS—sagittal, transverse, right oblique, and left oblique.
  - The mobility of the uterus should be evaluated—normal, reduced, or fixed ("question mark sign")
  - Describe the presence of endometrioma, if any, their size, and position.
  - The description of endometrioma should be based on the International Ovarian Tumor Analysis (IOTA) classification.
- *Features to look for:* The IDEA protocol lists a number of soft markers such as site-specific tenderness and fixed ovaries where we can assume the likelihood of suspected adhesion or superficial peritoneal endometriosis **(Box 1)**. These features include:
  - Ovarian endometriomas
  - DIE
  - *Adhesions:* If the structures are fixed despite probe pressure or abdominal palpation, adhesion can be suspected. If there is pelvic fluid in pouch of Douglas (POD), fine strands of tissue can also be visualized between uterus

TABLE 1: Steps of dynamic ultrasonography.

Steps	Procedure
First	Routine evaluation of uterus and adnexa (+ sonographic signs of adenomyosis/presence or absence of endometrioma)
Second	Evaluation of transvaginal sonographic "soft markers" (i.e., site-specific tenderness and ovarian mobility)
Third	Assessment of status of POD using real-time ultrasound-based "sliding sign"
Fourth	Assessment for DIE nodules in anterior and posterior compartments

(POD: pouch of Douglas; DIE: deep infiltrating endometriosis)

> **BOX 1:** Dynamic ultrasonography sequence of assessment for IDEA.
>
> - *Bowel:*
>   - Anterior rectum
>   - Rectosigmoid junction
>   - Sigmoid colon
> - *Uterus:*
>   - Morphology (using MUSA statement)
>   - Sliding sign for pouch of Douglas obliteration
> - *Adnexa:*
>   - Endometriomas or other ovarian masses (using IOTA statement)
>   - Mobility, including "kissing" ovaries sign
> - *Anterior compartment:*
>   - Bladder
>   - Ureterovesical junction
>   - Ureters
>   - +/− transabdominal ultrasound for kidneys
> - *Posterior compartment:*
>   - Posterior vaginal fornix
>   - Rectovaginal septum
>   - Uterosacral ligaments
> - *Site-specific tenderness:*
>   - Uterus and cervix
>   - Adnexa
>   - Uterosacral ligaments
>   - Pouch of Douglas
>
> (IOTA: International Ovarian Tumor Analysis; MUSA: morphological uterus sonographic assessment)

and adnexa. Such adhesions may distort the architecture of fallopian tubes and disease may complicate. Thus, such hydro/hematosalpinx or peritoneal cysts should also be noted.

- *Measurements:* These measurements include:
  - Size of ovarian endometriomas
  - Depth of DIE lesions
  - Number of adhesions

With the help of a sliding sign (TVS-based), the next thing is to assess POD to rule out various uterine versions. By placing a gentle pressure on cervix, we assess the ease through which the anterior wall of the rectum glides against retrocervical and posterior vaginal wall **(Figs. 3A and B)**.

The next step is to assess the fundus of uterus, which is done by palpating abdominally, balloting the uterus between hand and probe. If either of the areas, whether retrocervical or fundal, does not glide well, it will reflect a negative sliding sign, which suggests POD obliteration.

The next step is to search for DIE nodules in the anterior and posterior compartments **(Fig. 4)**. For the anterior compartment, the probe is placed in the anterior fornix of vagina over a partially filled bladder. For the posterior compartment, the probe is placed over the posterior fornix of vagina and slowly withdrawn to look for nodules.

Bladder: The assessment is done into four zones—trigonal zone, bladder base, bladder dome, and extra-abdominal bladder. The nodules have to be measured in three orthogonal planes. Bladder DIE is diagnosed only if muscularis of the bladder wall is affected; a lesion affecting serosa will represent superficial disease.

Uterovesical region: The TVS probe is placed in the anterior fornix, and the uterus is balloted between the probe and one hand of operator placed over the suprapubic region. Adhesion between the bladder and the anterior uterine wall in the anterior pelvic compartment can be visualized to check for a sliding sign. But such a sign cannot be discriminated with adhesion of previous cesarean section from endometriosis.

Ureters: First, we need to identify the urethra in the sagittal plane and move the probe toward the lateral pelvic wall. Dilatation of ureter due to endometriosis is caused by stricture, and distance from distal ureteric orifice to stricture should be measured.

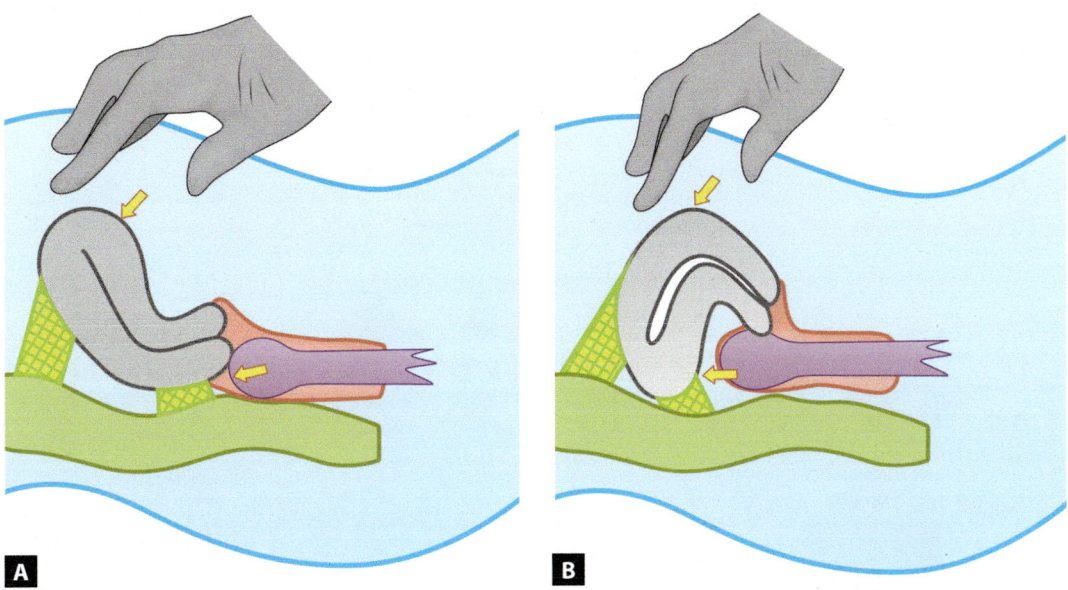

Figs. 3A and B: Assessment via sliding sign in anteverted and retroverted uterus.

With a known case of DIE, kidney assessment is done for ureteral stricture as most of such DIE are asymptomatic. With renal pelvic assessment, we categorize the degree of hydronephrosis so as to assess the need of stenting to maintain renal functioning.

Posterior compartment: For DIE, we need to ascertain the number, location, and size of nodules affecting USLs, posterior vaginal fornix, anterior rectosigmoid junction, and sigmoid colon.

Rectovaginal septum: The location to look for a DIE nodule in the rectovaginal space below the line passing along the lower border of the posterior lip of the cervix under the peritoneum.

Vaginal wall: Posterior vaginal fornix DIE is suspected if the area is thickened in the hypoechoic layer of the vaginal wall.

Rectovaginal nodules: Hourglass-shaped or diablo-like nodules occur when DIE lesions in the posterior vaginal fornix extend into the anterior rectal wall. These lesions will be partially fixed in the anterior rectal wall and partially in the posterior vaginal fornix.

Uterosacral ligaments: Place the TVS probe in the posterior vaginal fornix toward the midline in the sagittal plane after which the operator sweeps the probe inferolaterally to the cervix. These lesions can be seen as nothing but thickness in USL and can be measured in transverse plane at the insertion of the ligament on the cervix.

Rectum, rectosigmoid junction, and sigmoid: A very common site for such DIE lesions, they can present either as an isolation or can be multifocal or multicentric. Such lesions may appear on bowel as narrowing of lumen or thickening in hypoechoic muscularis propria or as hypoechoic nodules. Sometimes, such multiple nodules over the lumen may present as retraction or adhesions, giving an image of an Indian headdress or Moose Antler sign. A severe retraction of lumen may appear as pulling sleeve sign. A DIE nodule with progressive narrowing presents as comet sign **(Figs. 5A to F)**.

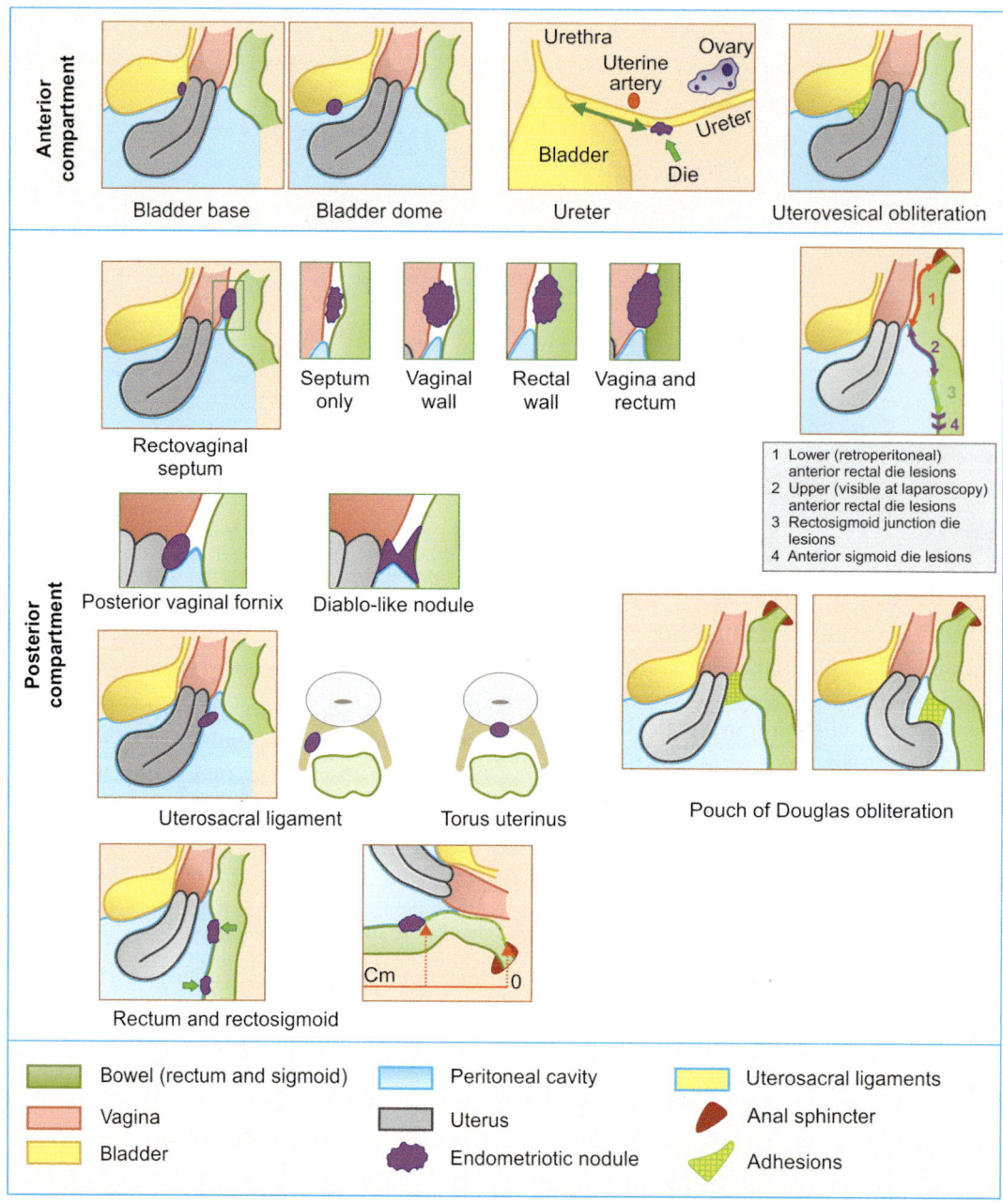

Fig. 4: Anterior and posterior compartments of the bladder.

- *Interpretation:* The IDEA protocol provides a standardized system for interpreting the findings of TVS for endometriosis. This system is based on the severity of the disease, the extent of the disease, and the presence or absence of adhesions.

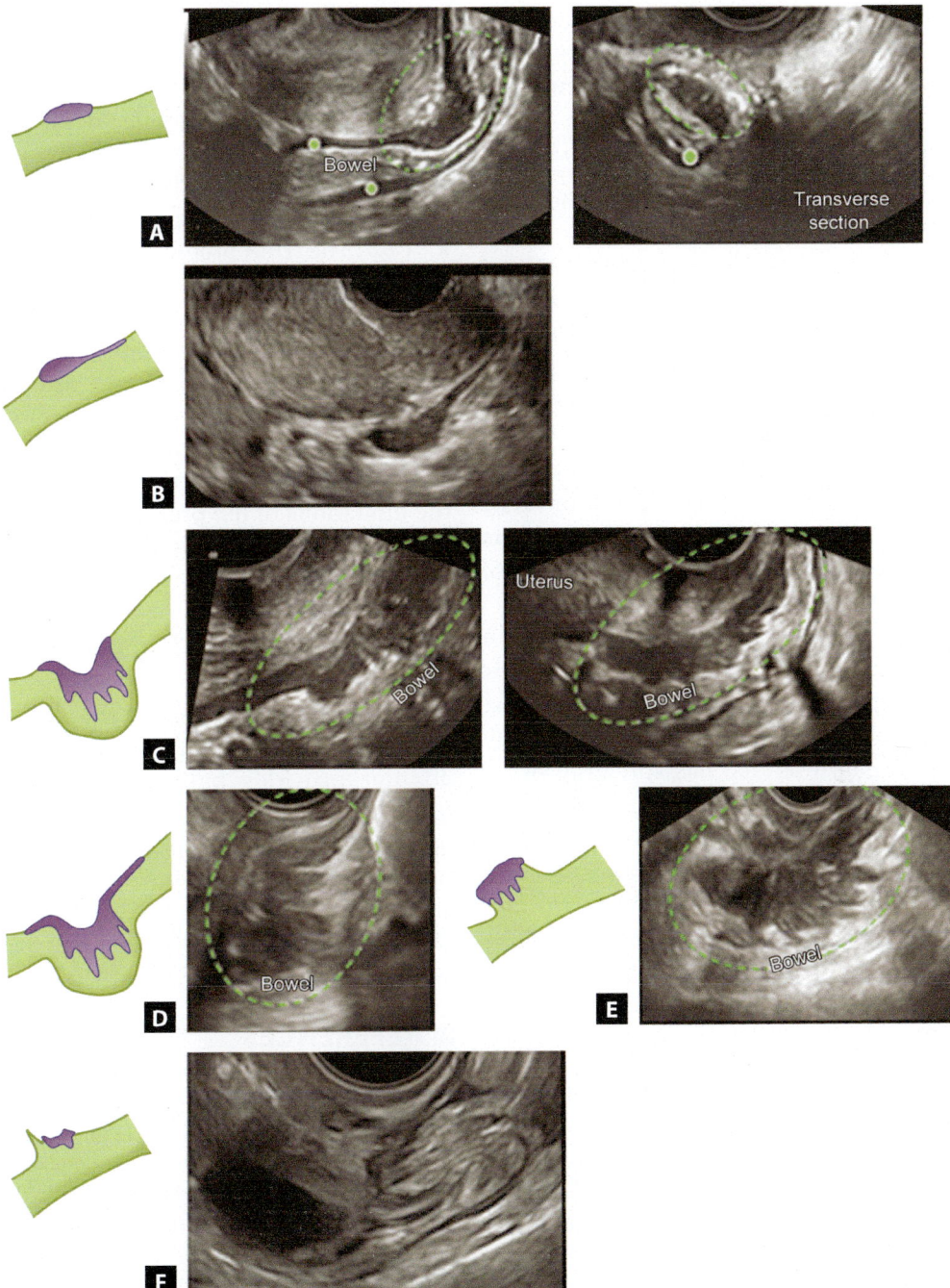

Figs. 5A to F: Drawing and sonographic representation of bowel deep infiltrating endometriosis. (A) DIE nodule with regular outline (absence of spikes); (B) Comet sign nodule with progressive narrowing; (C) Nodule with prominent spikes towards lumen (Indian headdress/Mosse Antler sign); (D) Nodule with both B and C; (E) Prominent spikes to lumen with extrinsic retraction (pulling sleeve sign); (F) Only extrinsic retraction.

The IDEA protocol has helped the clinicians by being a valuable tool via detecting and characterizing endometriosis.

Benefits of IDEA Protocol

Some of the specific advantages of the IDEA protocol are as follows:
- *Increased sensitivity:* The IDEA protocol has been shown to be more sensitive than standard TVS for the detection of endometriosis. This means that it is more likely to detect endometriosis, even if it is mild or early stage.
- *Improved specificity:* The IDEA protocol has also been shown to have improved specificity than standard TVS. This means that it is less likely to misdiagnose endometriosis as another condition.
- *More comprehensive evaluation:* The IDEA protocol evaluates the entire pelvis for signs of endometriosis and not just the ovaries. This can help to identify endometriosis that has spread to other areas, such as the bowel or bladder.
- *Standardized approach:* The IDEA protocol is a standardized approach to endometriosis imaging. This means that all clinicians who use the protocol will be using the same methods, which can help to improve the accuracy of diagnosis and the consistency of care.

Limitations of the IDEA protocol: The IDEA protocol is a valuable tool for clinicians who are managing women with endometriosis, but it is not without its limitations. Some of the issues that have been raised about IDEA imaging include the following:
- *Interobserver variability:* The IDEA protocol is a complex protocol, and it can be difficult for different clinicians to achieve the same level of accuracy when using it. This can lead to variability in the interpretation of images, which can impact the accuracy of diagnosis.
- *Technical limitations:* The IDEA protocol relies on the use of high-quality ultrasound equipment. In some settings, the equipment may not be up to the standard required to perform IDEA imaging accurately.
- *Cost:* The IDEA protocol is a more expensive imaging protocol than standard TVS. This can be a barrier to its use in some settings.

Despite these limitations, the IDEA protocol is an affordable and important too; for clinicians who are managing women with endometriosis. It is important to be aware of the limitations of the protocol, but it is also important to recognize its potential benefits.

CONCLUSION

The IDEA consensus for the diagnosis of endometriosis provides noninvasive, more accurate diagnosis of the degree of endometriosis severity. The four-step system adapter provides patients comfort and optimizes efficiency. It is true how such an approach requires an expert ultrasonologist; nevertheless, a novice sonologist doing TVS should know about the above approach to clinch the diagnosis and further manage the patient efficiently.

REFERENCES

1. Guerriero S, Ajossa S, Pagliuca M, Borzacchelli A, Deiala F, Springer S, et al. Advances in Imaging for Assessing Pelvic Endometriosis. Diagnostics (Basel). 2022;12(12):2960.
2. Lee SY, Koo YJ, Lee DH. Classification of endometriosis. Yeungnam Univ J Med. 2021; 38(1):10-8.
3. Tsamantioti ES, Mahdy H. (2023). Endometriosis. [online] In: StatPearls [Internet]. Treasure Island (FL): StatPearls Publishing; 2023.
4. Guerriero S, Condous G, van den Bosch T, Valentin L, Leone FP, Van Schoubroeck D,

et al. Systematic approach to sonographic evaluation of the pelvis in women with suspected endometriosis, including terms, definitions and measurements: A consensus opinion from the International Deep Endometriosis Analysis (IDEA) group. Ultrasound Obstet Gynecol. 2016; 48(3): 318-32.

5. Chen-Dixon K, Uzuner C, Mak J, Condous G. Effectiveness of ultrasound for endometriosis diagnosis. Curr Opin Obstet Gynecol. 2022; 34(5):324-31.

6. Leonardi M, Condous G. How to perform an ultrasound to diagnose endometriosis. Australas J Ultrasound Med. 2018;21(2): 61-9.

CHAPTER 6

Medical Management of Endometriosis

Kalyan B Barmade, Manisha K Barmade, Anand B Barmade

■ INTRODUCTION

The medical management of endometriosis is directed toward controlling pain and suppression of the hormonally active endometriotic tissue.[1] Endometriosis-related pain affects quality of life (QoL); and leads to cause of hospitalization, impairment of different aspects of health-related QoL, and high economic burden to women with endometriosis. Endometriosis pain usually arises from tissue damage at the site of lesions, and its severity may be correlated with the depth of infiltration of endometriosis; it rarely arises from nerve injury leading to neuropathic pain. There are different treatment modalities for relieving endometriosis-associated pain, including medical therapy, surgical interventions, and acupuncture.[2]

■ HORMONAL

- *Combined oral contraceptives:* The combined oral contraceptive pill (COCP) is widely used, although the evidence for its efficacy is limited with insufficient evidence.[3]
- *Progesterone-containing contraceptives:*
    - *Oral or injectable:* Randomized, controlled trial data to support the use of oral progestin-only treatment for pelvic pain associated with endometriosis and for suppressing the anatomic extent of endometriotic lesions.[4] Some of the progestins that have been studies and used in the treatment of endometriosis include cyproterone acetate, dienogest, dydrogesterone, gestrinone, lynestrenol, medroxyprogesterone acetate, megestrol acetate, and norethindrone acetate. Injectable progesterone offers the added advantage of better compliance by avoiding daily administration and erratic gastrointestinal absorption.[1]
- *Implant:* Etonogestrel implant, containing 68 mg etonogestrel that is slowly released for up to 3 years, provides an alternative way of delivering progestogens. It is a subcutaneous progestogen-releasing device which is helpful in decrease in pelvic pain with etonogestrel implants in patients suffering from endometriosis.[5]
- *Levonorgestrel-containing intrauterine system (LNG-IUS):* LNG-IUS is a T-shaped device that contains 52 mg of levonorgestrel, which releases 20 µg of hormone per day over a 5-year period. Several studies have suggested that LNG-IUS is effective as postoperative maintenance therapy

also to reduce the risk of recurrence of pain symptoms and endometrioma. Many cohort studies compare pain relief and recurrence prevention are similar to those of combined oral contraceptives or dienogest.[6,1]

- *Selective progesterone receptor modulators:*
  - *Mifepristone:* Moderate-quality evidence shows that mifepristone relieves dysmenorrhea (painful periods) and also relieves dyspareunia (pain during sexual intercourse). However, amenorrhea (absence of menstrual periods) and hot flushes are common side effects of mifepristone. 90% had amenorrhea, and 24% had hot flushes.[7]
  - *Ulipristal acetate:* Ulipristal acetate (ulipristal) is a selective progesterone receptor modulator (SPRM) that acts as an antagonist and partial agonist, preventing progesterone from binding its receptor.[8] It may have little effect of progestogenic activity on endometrium which may be helpful in relieving pain.[9]
- *Gonadotrophin-releasing hormone agonists:*
  - *Leuprolide acetate* reduces endometriotic lesions and improve pelvic pain/tenderness, dysmenorrhea, and dyspareunia. It can be advisable to use for a maximum duration of 6 months. It is administered either as a monotherapy or in combination with norethindrone acetate to reduce bone mineral density loss.[10]
  - *Nafarelin:* Nafarelin, a gonadotropin-releasing hormone agonist, has been shown to be effective in the treatment of endometriosis. Side effects most commonly include those associated with estrogen deprivation[11] so can be used judiciously.

■ NONHORMONAL

- *Nonsteroidal anti-inflammatory drugs (NSAIDS):* NSAIDS are widely used as first line in mild-to-moderate cases but has lack of high-quality evidence, does not support the use of NSAIDs, despite their current widespread use.[1,12]
- *Aromatase inhibitors (AIs):* The use of AIs in the treatment of endometriosis was based on the evidence of aromatase activity in ectopic endometrial lesions, and the relationship between the presence of extrauterine endometrial tissue and serum estrogen levels. Aromatase activity is absent in normal human endometrium and is increased in endometriosis. It was demonstrated that extrauterine endometrial tissue is a source of estrogens. Moreover, estrogens stimulate synthesis of prostaglandin E2 (PGE2), which is a potent inducer of aromatase activity in endometrium. This is the underlying mechanism that triggers the virtuous cycle leading to the new growth of ectopic endometrial tissue. The use of aromatase inhibitors in the treatment of endometriosis is supposed to stop this virtuous cycle.[13] can be given in continuous manner for long-term treatment modality.
- *Danazol:* The observation that hyperandrogenic states (an excess of male hormone) induce atrophy of the endometrium. The efficacy of danazol is based on its ability to produce a high-androgen/low-estrogen environment (a pseudomenopause), which result in an improvement in painful symptoms but its use is limited by the occurrence of androgenic side effects.[14]

NEWER ADVANCES

- *Cabergoline:* Dopamine and its agonists, such as cabergoline, promote VEGF receptor-2 endocytosis in endothelial cells; therefore, VEGF-VEGFR-2 binding is prevented and neoangiogenesis is decreased. It has been found that daily treatment with cabergoline suppresses cell proliferation and VEGF-mediated angiogenesis, thereby helping in regression of endometriotic lesions. So, cabergoline can be a novel drug for the treatment of chronic pelvic pain due to endometriosis.[15]

- *Gonadotrophin-releasing hormone antagonists:* Elagolix, a nonpeptide, small-molecule gonadotropin-releasing hormone (GnRH) receptor antagonist, is the first new oral therapy to be approved for the treatment of endometriosis-associated pain. Modulation of estradiol with elagolix is dose-dependent and ranges from partial to full suppression. Clinical evidence has shown that elagolix at both approved doses (150 mg once daily and 200 mg twice daily) is effective for reducing symptoms of pelvic pain (dysmenorrhea, nonmenstrual pelvic pain, and dyspareunia), improving QoL, and decreasing use of rescue analgesics (nonsteroidal anti-inflammatory drugs and/or opioids).[16]

REFERENCES

1. Rafique S, Decherney AH. Medical management of endometriosis. Clin Obstet Gynecol. 2017;60(3):485-96. doi: 10.1097/GRF.0000000000000292.
2. Samy A, Taher A, Sileem SA, Abdelhakim AM, Fathi M, Haggag H, et al. Medical therapy options for endometriosis related pain, which is better? A systematic review and network meta-analysis of randomized controlled trials. J Gynecol Obstet Hum Reprod. 2021;50(1):101798. doi: 10.1016/j.jogoh.2020.101798.
3. Brown J, Crawford TJ, Datta S, Prentice A. Oral contraceptives for pain associated with endometriosis. Cochrane Database Syst Rev. 2018;5(5):CD001019. doi: 10.1002/14651858.
4. Casper RF. Progestin-only pills may be a better first-line treatment for endometriosis than combined estrogen-progestin contraceptive pills. Fertil Steril. 2017;107(3):533-6. doi: 10.1016/j.fertnstert.2017.01.003.
5. Niu X, Luo Q, Wang C, Zhu L, Huang L. Effects of etonogestrel implants on pelvic pain and menstrual flow in women suffering from adenomyosis or endometriosis: Results from a prospective, observational study. Medicine (Baltimore). 2021;100(6):e24597. doi: 10.1097/MD.0000000000024597.
6. Kim HY, Song SY, Jung SH, Song HJ, Lee M, Lee KH, et al. Long-term efficacy and safety of levonorgestrel-releasing intrauterine system as a maintenance treatment for endometriosis. Medicine (Baltimore). 2022;101(10):e29023. doi: 10.1097/MD.0000000000029023.
7. Fu J, Song H, Zhou M, Zhu H, Wang Y, Chen H, et al. Progesterone receptor modulators for endometriosis. Cochrane Database Syst Rev. 2017;7(7):CD009881. doi: 10.1002/14651858.CD009881.pub2.
8. Bressler LH, Bernardi LA, Snyder MA, Wei JJ, Bulun S. Treatment of endometriosis-related chronic pelvic pain with Ulipristal Acetate and associated endometrial changes. HSOA J Reprod Med Gynaecol Obstet. 2017;2:008. doi: 10.24966/RMGO-2574/100008.
9. De Milliano I, Van Hattum D, Ket JCF, Huirne JAF, Hehenkamp WJK. Endometrial changes during ulipristal acetate use: A systematic review. Eur J Obstet Gynecol Reprod Biol. 2017;214:56-64. doi: 10.1016/j.ejogrb.2017.04.042.
10. Swayzer DV, Gerriets V. (2023). Leuprolide. Treasure Island (FL): StatPearls Publishing; 2022. Available from: https://www.ncbi.nlm.nih.gov/books/NBK551662/. [Last accessed June, 2023].

11. Hull ME, Barbieri RL. Nafarelin in the treatment of endometriosis. Dose management. Gynecol Obstet Invest. 1994;37(4):263-4. doi: 10.1159/000292574.
12. Brown J, Crawford TJ, Allen C, Hopewell S, Prentice A. Nonsteroidal anti-inflammatory drugs for pain in women with endometriosis. Cochrane Database Syst Rev. 2017;1(1):CD004753. doi: 10.1002/14651858.CD004753.pub4.
13. Słopień R, Męczekalski B. Aromatase inhibitors in the treatment of endometriosis. Prz Menopauzalny. 2016;15(1):43-7. doi: 10.5114/pm.2016.58773. Epub 2016 Mar 29. PMID: 27095958; PMCID: PMC4828508.
14. Selak V, Farquhar C, Prentice A, Singla A. Danazol for pelvic pain associated with endometriosis. Cochrane Database Syst Rev. 2000;(2):CD000068. doi: 10.1002/14651858.CD000068. Update in: Cochrane Database Syst Rev. 2001;(4):CD000068.
15. Does cabergoline help in decreasing chronic pelvic pain due to endometriosis compared to medroxyprogesterone acetate? A Prospective Randomized Study. J South Asian Fed Obstet Gynecol. 2018;10(3):167-9.
16. Leyland N, Estes SJ, Lessey BA, Advincula AP, Taylor HS. A clinician's guide to the treatment of endometriosis with elagolix. J Womens Health (Larchmt). 2021;30(4):569-78. doi: 10.1089/jwh.2019.8096.

Surgical Management of Endometriosis

Ankita Bansal Goyal, Aruna Suman

■ INTRODUCTION

Surgical management is usually indicated for the correction of pain, infertility, and other possible symptoms according to the extent of the disease, or when the hormonal treatments are failing to provide symptomatic relief in early stages. Surgery is usually associated with significant improvement in pain management scores and restoration of fertility as compared to hormonal treatment in many cases of advanced disease.[1]

Surgical management of endometriosis requires a multimodal approach and individualization according to the clinical presentation, severity and extent of the disease, previous treatment received and future fertility requirements. Laparoscopy is usually preferred over conventional laparotomy because although both the techniques are equally effective, laparoscopy is associated with quicker recovery, less postoperative morbidity, pain, and fewer postoperative adhesions. Laparotomy is usually reserved for the advanced cases where laparoscopy is not possible.

Laparoscopy surgery can be done for both diagnostic and therapeutic purposes. However, surgical management should be done at the time of diagnosis only to avoid repeat surgery to the patient, provided the preoperative consent was obtained.[2]

The surgical treatment is usually guided by careful patient assessment, including meticulous recording of symptoms, physical findings on examination, and preoperative imaging.

The goal of the surgery should be restoration of normal anatomy with the excision of all visible endometriotic spots and removal of all possible adhesions.[3]

The surgery can be conservative or definitive (radical surgery including hysterectomy and bilateral oophorectomy).

■ CONSERVATIVE SURGERIES

Resection of implants:[4]
- Resection of implants requires good surgical skills and through knowledge of anatomy.
- Implant should be localized and incision should be given in the peritoneum near to it.
- Peritoneum should be the adequately mobilized over the organs; it may require opening of retroperitoneum.
- Sometimes, implants are on the vital structure which may need opening of avascular spaces of pelvis (pararectal, paravesical, vesicovaginal, rectovaginal, and the space of retzius).
- If a lesion overlies the ureter, it can be mobilized with blunt dissection along

with its pelvic course, pushing and spreading just adjacent to the ureter rather than directly on it.
- Excise the lesion and surrounding peritoneum with sharp scissors, ultrasonic energy, or monopolar cautery.

Peritoneal endometriosis: Peritoneal lesions can be removed by surgical excisions with electrocautery, scissors, or laser ablation (CO_2 laser, potassium-titanyl-phosphate laser, or argon laser).[5] Some surgeons claim that CO_2 laser is superior because of minimal thermal damage; however, no evidence is available to show the superiority of one technique over the other.[6] Surgical excision is considered equally effective to ablation with added advantage of tissue availability for histopathological analysis and confirmation of endometriosis.[5]

Ovarian endometriosis:[7,8]
- Superficial ovarian lesions can be vaporized.
- Ovarian endometrioma can be managed with either cystectomy or drainage and ablation of the cyst wall.
- *Cystectomy:* Endometrioma is drained and the cyst wall is excised from the ovarian cortex trying to preserve maximum number of follicles.
- During drainage and ablation procedure followed by drainage of endometrioma, cyst wall is inspected for intracystic lesions and is vaporized to destroy the mucosal lining of the cyst.
- Because of the evidence of less recurrence of endometrioma and symptoms of dysmenorrhea, the European Society of Human Reproduction and Embryology (ESHRE) recommends cystectomy over drainage and ablation.

- In cases of very large endometrioma where excision is technically difficult without removing a large part of the ovary, a three-step procedure [marsupialization and rinsing followed by hormonal treatment with gonadotropin-releasing hormone (GnRH) analogs and cyst wall electrocoagulation or laser vaporization 3 months later] can be considered.

Deep endometriosis:[1,3,9]
- Management of deep lesions are usually difficult due to its extensive nature and multifocal involvement.
- It should be done only after careful evaluation of the patient, preoperative imaging, and proper counseling of the patient about the possible complications.
- It should be carried out in tertiary center with multidisciplinary approach.
- Surgery should be carried out only for the symptomatic cases. Asymptomatic cases should not be operated unless there is significant ureteric obstruction leading to asymptomatic loss of renal function.
- Complete excision of the lesion should be the aim.
- If there is involvement of the bladder, it should be removed; and primary closure of the bladder wall should be done.
- Ureteric lesions should be excised after stenting. In presence of intrinsic lesions and significant obstruction, segmental excision should be done with end-to-end anastomosis.
- Surgical excision of deep rectovaginal and rectosigmoidal endometriosis is difficult and can be associated with major complications such as bowel perforations with resulting peritonitis. It is debated whether this type of endometriosis is best treated by shaving, conservative excision, or resection anastomosis.

Interruption of pelvic nerve pathways:[10,11]
- Surgical interruption of pelvic nerve pathway has been suggested as an additional procedure to conservative surgeries.
- Two techniques have been suggested—laparoscopic uterine nerve ablation (LUNA), and presacral neurectomy (PSN)
- Based on the systemic review, LUNA should not be combined with conservative surgeries and it has shown no additional benefit.
- PSN is effective as an additional procedure, but it requires a high degree of surgical skills and is associated with increased adverse effects such as bleeding, constipation, and urinary urgency.

Outcomes of conservative surgery:[12,13]
- Outcome is usually influenced by many psychological factors such as personality, depression, and marital and sexual problems.
- It is difficult to objectify the outcome due to several variables such as the extent of disease, operators experience, and associated comorbidities.
- The extent and duration of the therapeutic benefit of surgery for endometriosis-related pain are poorly defined; and the expected benefit is operator dependent.

Prevention of recurrence after conservative surgical treatment:[14-16]

Addition of postoperative hormonal therapy is usually given postsurgery for two main reasons:
1. Short-term postoperative hormonal therapy (6 months) could improve the operative outcome through their effect on residual endometriosis.
2. Long-term hormonal therapy could be prescribed for secondary prevention, i.e., suppression of ovarian function can prevent emergence of new lesions.

Based on available evidence, there is no role of short-term use of hormonal treatment to improve the outcome of conservative surgery; hence, it is not recommended by the ESHRE.

The ESHRE guidelines recommend the use of postoperative hormonal therapy for two indications:
1. After cystectomy in women not immediately seeking fertility.
2. For secondary prevention of endometriosis-associated dysmenorrhea for at least 18–20 months.

Radical surgery, oophorectomy, and hysterectomy:[16]
- Usually indicated in severe situations
- Along with radical surgery, all visible endometriotic spots should be removed.
- Complete surgery at young age should be considered only in most severe and recurrent cases.

REFERENCES

1. Abbott JA, Hawe J, Clayton RD, Garry R. The effects and effectiveness of laparoscopic excision of endometriosis: a prospective study with 2-5 year follow-up. Hum Reprod. 2003;18(9):1922-7.
2. Redwine DB, Wright JT. Laparoscopic treatment of complete obliteration of the cul-de-sac associated with endometriosis: long-term follow-up of en bloc resection. Fertil Steril. 2001;76(2):358-65.
3. Fedele L, Bianchi S, Zanconato G, Bettoni G, Gotsch F. Long-term follow-up after conservative surgery for rectovaginal endometriosis. Am J Obstet Gynecol. 2004;190(4):1020-4.
4. Koninckx PR, Timmermans B, Meuleman C, Penninckx F. Complications of CO_2-laser endoscopic excision of deep endometriosis. Hum Reprod. 1996;11(10):2263-8.
5. Dunselman GA, Vermeulen N, Becker C, Calhaz-Jorge C, D'Hooghe T, De Bie B, et al;

European Society of Human Reproduction and Embryology. ESHRE guideline: management of women with endometriosis. Hum Reprod. 2014;29(3):400-12.
6. Donnez J, Nisolle M, Gillet N, Smets M, Bassil S, Casanas-Roux F. Large ovarian endometriomas. Hum Reprod. 1996;11(3): 641-6.
7. Chapron C, Chopin N, Borghese B, Foulot H, Dousset B, Vacher-Lavenu MC, et al. Deeply infiltrating endometriosis: pathogenetic implications of the anatomical distribution. Hum Reprod. 2006;21(7):1839-45.
8. Proctor ML, Latthe PM, Farquhar CM, Khan KS, Johnson NP. Surgical interruption of pelvic nerve pathways for primary and secondary dysmenorrhoea. Cochrane Database Syst Rev. 2005;2005(4):CD001896.
9. Candiani GB, Fedele L, Vercellini P, Bianchi S, Di Nola G. Presacral neurectomy for the treatment of pelvic pain associated with endometriosis: a controlled study. Am J Obstet Gynecol. 1992;167(1):100-3.
10. Sutton CJ, Ewen SP, Whitelaw N, Haines P. Prospective, randomized, double-blind, controlled trial of laser laparoscopy in the treatment of pelvic pain associated with minimal, mild, and moderate endometriosis. Fertil Steril. 1994;62(4):696-700.
11. Vercellini P, Crosignani PG, Abbiati A, Somigliana E, Viganò P, Fedele L. The effect of surgery for symptomatic endometriosis: the other side of the story. Hum Reprod Update. 2009;15(2):177-88.
12. Yap C, Furness S, Farquhar C. Pre and post operative medical therapy for endometriosis surgery. Cochrane Database Syst Rev. 2004; 2004(3):CD003678. Update in: Cochrane Database Syst Rev. 2020;11:CD003678.
13. Bianchi S, Busacca M, Agnoli B, Candiani M, Calia C, Vignali M. Effects of 3 month therapy with danazol after laparoscopic surgery for stage III/IV endometriosis: a randomized study. Hum Reprod. 1999;14(5):1335-7.
14. Parazzini F, Fedele L, Busacca M, Falsetti L, Pellegrini S, Venturini PL, et al. Post-surgical medical treatment of advanced endometriosis: results of a randomized clinical trial. Am J Obstet Gynecol. 1994; 171(5):1205-7.
15. Lefebvre G, Allaire C, Jeffrey J, Vilos G, Arneja J, Birch C, et al; Clinical Practice Gynaecology Committee and Executive Committeee and Council, Society of Obstetricians and Gynaecologists of Canada. SOGC clinical guidelines. Hysterectomy. J Obstet Gynaecol Can. 2002;24(1):37-61; quiz 74-6.
16. Namnoum AB, Hickman TN, Goodman SB, Gehlbach DL, Rock JA. Incidence of symptom recurrence after hysterectomy for endometriosis. Fertil Steril. 1995;64(5): 898-902.

CHAPTER 8

Endometriosis and Assisted Reproduction Technology

T Ramani Devi, C Archana Devi

■ INTRODUCTION

Endometriosis is a chronic inflammatory disorder, which is estrogen dependent and progesterone resistant, characterized by the presence of endometrial glands and stroma outside the endometrial cavity.[1]

Almost every woman has retrograde menstruation and menstrual debris reach the peritoneal cavity every month but why only some women develop the enigmatic disease, endometriosis, is not known.

The incidence of endometriosis is found to be 1 in 10 women of reproductive age group and the Federation of Obstetric and Gynaecological Societies of India (FOGSI) good clinical Practice Recommendations (GCPR) 2016[2] also state the same. Among infertile women, 25–48% suffer from endometriosis.[3] 70% of women with chronic pelvic pain also suffer from endometriosis.[4] 5–7% of adolescent girls suffer from endometriosis. 40–60% of girls with severe dysmenorrhea have endometriosis.[5]

Hence, it may be viewed as a disease that starts in utero and spans the entire reproductive age group of women, even beyond menopause.

About 190 million women or even more, across the globe suffer from endometriosis according to the World Endometriosis Society. The Endometriosis Society of India quotes an incidence of 50 million and above in India.[6]

Endometriosis has two important implications in a woman's life. One is infertility and the other is severe pelvic pain. It is a challenging medical condition for the concerned physician, as the root cause for the pathogenesis of endometriosis is not hit by any mode of treatment. The diagnostic delay may be up to 6–7 years. This may be because earlier treatment was started after histological confirmation through laparoscopy. The concept of treating without histopathological confirmation has been endorsed by the World Endometriosis Society, the American Society for Reproductive Medicine (ASRM), the European Society of Human Reproduction and Embryology (ESHRE), the Society of Obstetricians and Gynaecologists of Canada (SOGC), and FOGSI.[7-11] Hence, there is an emerging role for medical management without histopathological evidence.

■ INCIDENCE

Endometriosis is an enigmatic disease affecting up to 10% of reproductive age group women. 25–50% of infertile women are likely to suffer from endometriosis and infertility is seen among 30–50% of women with endometriosis (Bulletti C et al., 2010).[12]

THEORIES ON PATHOGENESIS OF ENDOMETRIOSIS

Theories which explain the development of endometriosis include retrograde menstruation (Sampson, 1925), Coelomic Metaplasia (Meyer, 1924; Iwanoff, 1898; Lauche, 1923), Hormonal theory (Novak, 1931), Apoptosis suppression and alteration (Ferryman 1994, Taniguchi 2011), Genetics (Hadfield, 1994; Seli, 2003; Alberisen, 2013), Immune dysfunction (Semino, 1995), Oxidative stress and inflammation (Murphy, 1998) and Stem cells (Tsuji, 2008, Kato, 2012; Deane, 2013). There is no single universally accepted theory for the pathogenesis of endometriosis and it is evident that the presence of endometrial-like tissue outside the uterus causes chronic inflammatory reaction **(Fig. 1)**.

There are some polygenetic, polyepigenetic mechanisms in the development of endometriosis.[13] Endometriosis is a hereditary and a heterogeneous disease with many biochemical changes which are clonal in origin. The set of genetic and epigenetic mechanisms is transmitted at birth. This explains the hereditary aspects of the predisposition and endometriosis-associated changes in the endometrium, immunology, and placentation.

EPIDEMIOLOGICAL FACTORS AND MOLECULAR MECHANISMS INVOLVED IN ENDOMETRIOSIS DEVELOPMENT

Previous researchers have shown that endometriosis is prevalent after menarche

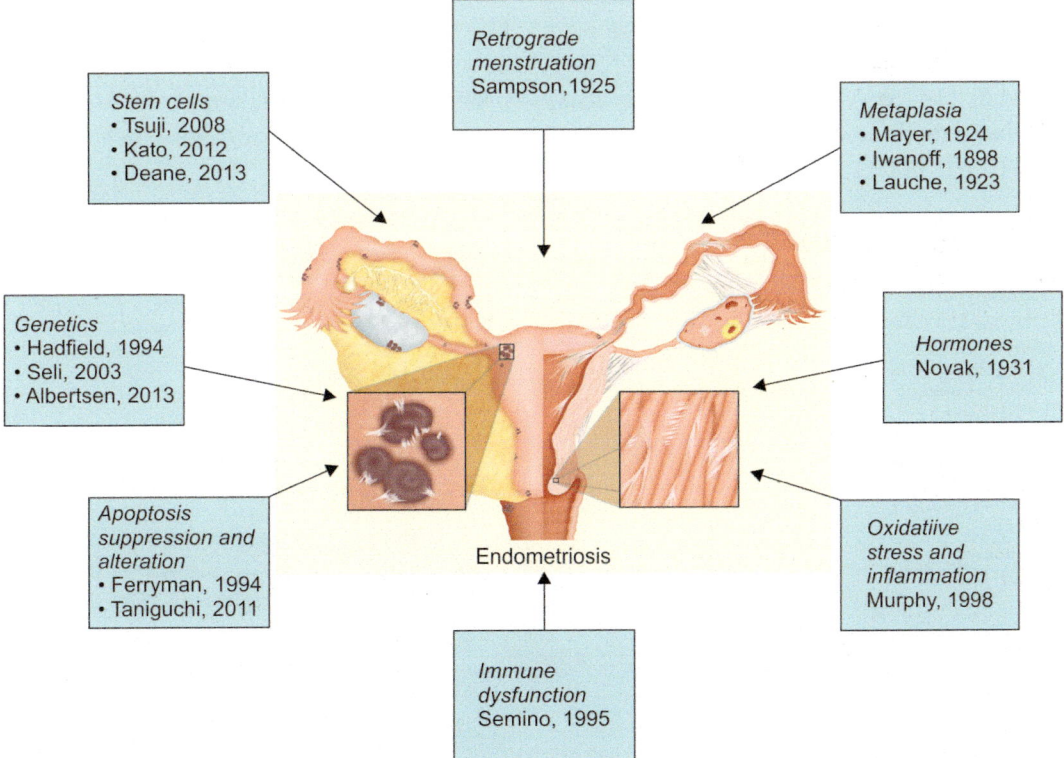

Fig. 1: Theories on pathogenesis of endometriosis.

(at the onset of thelarche) and dramatically decreases after menopause, which has led them to believe that the disorder is estrogen dependent.

Various epidemiological factors which drastically influence the development of endometriosis include early menarche, short menstrual cycle, increased duration of menstrual flow, and decreased parity.

Other constitutional factors include a positive family history (6.9 times higher incidence), consumption of alcohol, sedentary lifestyle, and inconsistent diet. Smoking has no effect.

MOLECULAR AND CELLULAR ALTERATIONS

There is altered steroid biosynthesis and receptor response, which includes increased $ER\beta$ expression, increased aromatase expression, perturbations in progesterone signal intermediates, $HOXA10$, $FOXA1$, $NF\text{-}kB$, Hic 5, $NCoR2$, and 17β-hydroxy steroid dehydrogenase 2 deficiencies. There is profound increase in the inflammatory factors such as overexpression of COX-2, and prostaglandins.

Increased peritoneal vascular endothelial growth factor (VEGF), overactive AKT, upregulated matrix metalloproteinases (MMP) expression, recruitment of Tie-2 expressing macrophages are few factors which contribute increased invasiveness and vascularization. Certain other inflammatory responses which trigger endometriosis include production of chemokines such as interleukin (IL)-8, monocyte chemotactic protein-1 (MCP1), RANTES (Regulated upon Activation, Normal T Cell Expressed and Presumably Secreted), Peritoneal IL6, tumor necrosis factor alpha (TNF-α), T helper (Th) 1 cytokines, antiapoptosis factor, recruitment of alternatively activated macrophages, engagement of nuclear factor kappa B (NF-kB)-dependent pathway, and accumulation of iron, and reactive oxygen species (ROS) production.[3] There is suppression of Th 2 and anti-inflammatory cytokines such as

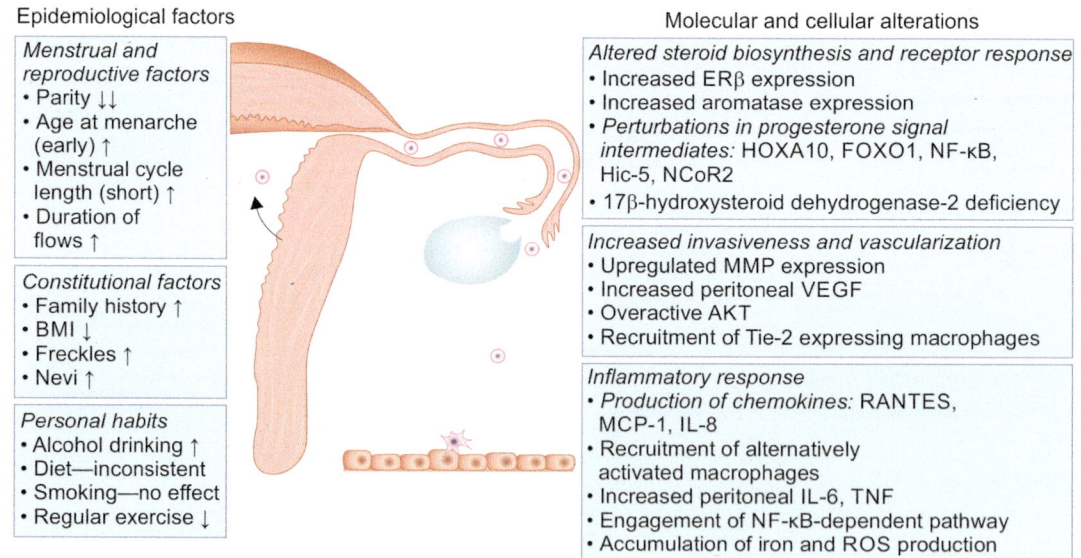

Fig. 2: Epidemiology of endometriosis and molecular and cellular alteration.

IL-4, IL-10, and IL-13; and P53 apoptosis induction. Understanding of the basic pathogenesis will help us to formulate the medical management.[14] This will help to plan the fertility treatment **(Fig. 2)**.

SYMPTOMS

Common symptoms of endometriosis are pain and infertility, and 20–25% of patients are asymptomatic **(Table 1)**.

CAUSES FOR INFERTILITY IN ENDOMETRIOSIS

Infertile women are six to eight times more likely to have endometriosis than fertile women.[15] Despite extensive research, no conclusive mechanism has been proposed to explain the association between endometriosis and infertility.

Various mechanisms proposed include:
- Distorted pelvic anatomy
- Altered utero tubal transport
- Endocrine and ovulatory abnormalities
- Altered peritoneal function
- Endometrium shows altered hormonal and cell-mediated functions

Decreased oocyte, embryo quality, and lowered number of blastomeres which get arrested by 72 hours.[16]

The harmful effects of increased inflammatory activity in the peritoneal cavity upon tubal function, oocytes, sperm and/or embryos are:
- Progesterone resistance in eutopic endometrium
- Decreased expression of integrins, *HOXA* genes, increased uterine NK cells, and production of immunoglobulins
- There are abnormalities in the molecular level such as defective steroidogenesis, increased aromatase activity and reduced progesterone formation. There is increased ROS, nitric oxide, and nitric oxide synthetase.

Donor eggs implant very well and eggs of suboptimal quality implanted in healthy women which showed oocytes are at fault rather than endometrium.

Following factors have to be taken into consideration for treatment of endometriosis: Age of the patient, associated tubal and male factor, symptoms, and duration of infertility. Current treatment options for fertility are expectant, medical, surgical, combination, and assisted reproduction technology (ART). Aim of treatment is to remove the implants, restore the anatomy, and improve the fecundity **(Fig. 3)**.

STAGING AND CLASSIFICATION FOR ENDOMETRIOSIS

Commonly used staging is the ASRM revised classification for endometriosis, which can grade the severity but this classification cannot predict the fertility outcome. Hence, there is a need for better classification and index which can predict the fertility outcome. Endometriosis fertility index is one such index which can predict the outcome of fertility based on history, r-ASRM scoring, and laparoscopic findings.

TABLE 1: Common symptoms of endometriosis.

Dysmenorrhea	60–80%
Chronic pelvic pain	40–50%
Deep dyspareunia	40–50%
Infertility	30–50%
Severe menstrual pain and irregular flow and /or premenstrual spotting	10–20%
Tenesmus, dyschezia, hematochezia, costiveness, or diarrhea	1–2%
Dysuria, pollakiuria, micro- or macroscopic hematuria	1–2%

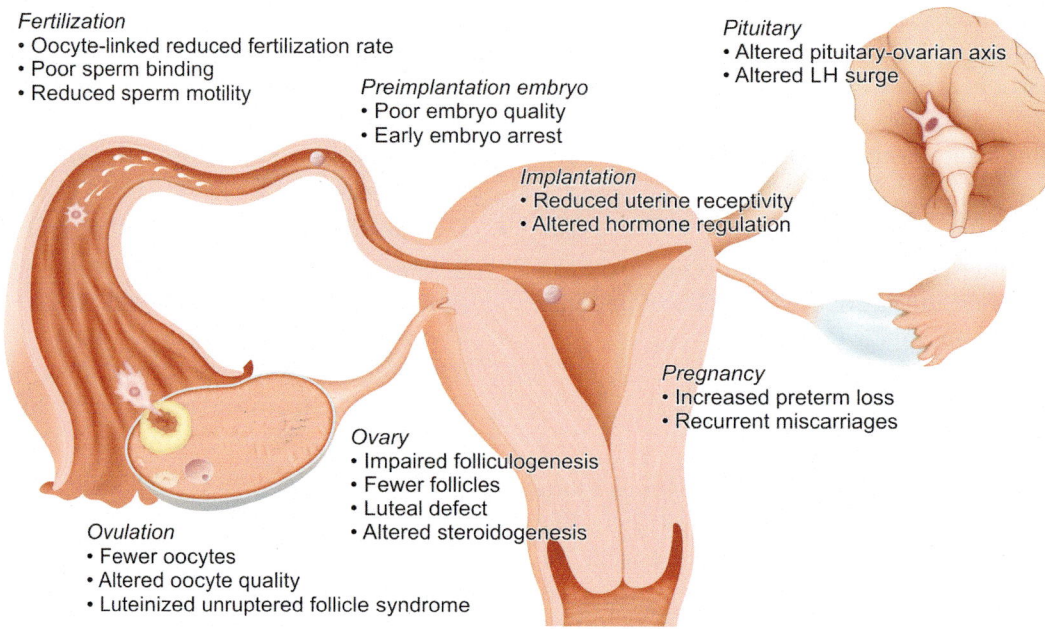

Fig. 3: Reasons for infertility in endometriosis.

ENDOMETRIOSIS FERTILITY INDEX

Endometriosis fertility index (EFI) is the first validated scoring system that is predictive of non-ART pregnancy following surgery, when the patient has functional gametes and uterus. Pregnancy rates decrease significantly with decreased ovarian reserve, which is especially a problem in older patients. It is also reflected in the EFI, which decreases over time if pregnancy does not occur in the first year or two following surgeries. EFI is graded as 10 points and this can predict the natural fertility or pregnancies following ovulation induction after surgery for endometriosis for a period of subsequent 2 years. Maximum pregnancies occur within first 12–18 months beyond which pregnancy rates are low. Patients with EFI score >7 can attempt spontaneous conception. Patients with EFI score of 5–6 can be given a trial of natural conception/ovulation induction conception for a short period. Patients with EFI score of <4 should be advised direct ART. Thus, EFI can be used as a guide for the clinicians and the patients to plan comprehensive mode of fertility treatment **(Figs. 4 and 5)**.[17]

MANAGEMENT OF ENDOMETRIOSIS-RELATED INFERTILITY

The clinical management of an infertile couple should take into account the age of the female, duration of infertility, male factor, duration of medical treatment, pelvic pain, and stage of endometriosis. Fertility among endometriosis can be improved by operative laparoscopy which can restore the normal pelvic anatomy. It should be suggested to women with endometriosis having infertility <33 years, as there is reduction in ovarian reserve beyond 35 years. Hence, following

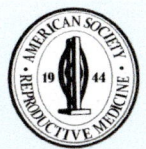

American Society for Reproductive Medicine
Revised Classification of Endometriosis

Patient's name_____ Date_____

Stage I (Minimal) — 1–5   Laparoscopy_____ Laparotomy_____ Photography_____
Stage II (Mild) — 6–15   Recommended treatment_____
Stage III (Moderate) — 16–40   _____
Stage IV (Severe) — >40
Total_____   Prognosis_____

	Endometriosis	<1 cm	1–3 cm	>3 cm
Peritoneum	Superficial	1	2	4
	Deep	2	4	6
Ovary	R Superficial	1	2	4
	Deep	4	16	20
	L Superficial	1	2	4
	Deep	4	16	20
	Posterior cul-de-sac obliteration	Partial		Complete
		4		40
	Adhesions	<1/3 enclosure	1/3–2/3 enclosure	>2/3 enclosure
Ovary	R Filmy	1	2	4
	Dense	4	8	16
	L Filmy	1	2	4
	Dense	4	8	16
Tube	R Filmy	1	2	4
	Dense	4*	8*	16
	L Filmy	1	2	4
	Dense	4*	8*	16

*If the fimbriated end of the fallopian tube is completely enclosed, change the point assignment to 16.
Denote appearance of superficial implant types as red [(R), red, red-pink, flamelike, vesicular blobs, clear vesicles], white [(W), opacifications, peritoneal defects, yellow-brown], or black [(B), black, hemosiderin deposits, blue]. Denote percent of total described as R___%, W___% and B___%. Total should equal 100%.

Additional endometriosis_____   Associated pathology: _____
_____   _____
_____   _____

To be used with normal tubes and ovaries   To be used with abnormal tubes and/or ovaries

Fig. 4: Staging and classification for endometriosis.

Endometriosis Fertility Index (EFI) Surgery Form

Least function (LF) score at conclusion of surgery

Score	Description
4 =	Normal
3 =	Mild dysfunction
2 =	Moderate dysfunction
1 =	Severe dysfunction
0 =	Absent or nonfunctional

	Left	Right
Fallopian tube		
Fimbria		
Ovary		

To calculate the LF score, add together the lowest score for the left side and the lowest score for the right side. If an ovary is absent on one side, the LF score is obtained by doubling the lowest score on the side with the ovary.

Lowest score: Left + Right = LF score

Endometriosis fertility index (EFI)

Historical factors			Surgical factors		
Factor	Description	Points	Factor	Description	Points
Age	If age is ≤ 35 years	2	LF score	If LF score = 7–8 (high score)	3
	If age is 36–39 years	1		If LF score = 4–6 (moderate score)	2
	If age is ≥ 40 years	0		If LF score = 1–3 (low score)	0
Years infertile	If years infertile is ≤ 3	2	AFS endometriosis score	If AFS endometriosis lesion score is < 16	1
	If years infertile is > 3	0		If AFS endometriosis lesion score is ≥ 16	0
Prior pregnancy	If there is a history of a prior pregnancy	1	AFS total score	If AFS total score is < 71	1
	If there is no history of prior pregnancy	0		If AFS total score is ≥ 71	0
Total historical factors			Total surgical factors		

EFI = Total historical factors + total surgical factors: Historical + Surgical = EFI score

A

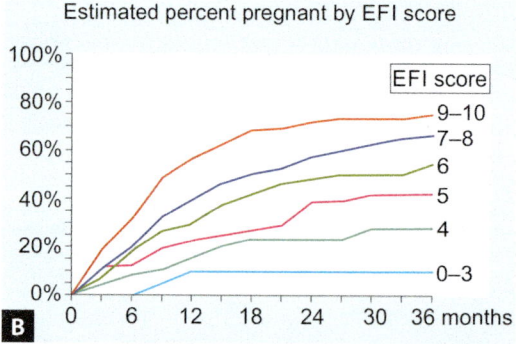

B

Figs. 5A and B: Fertility outcome and EFI scoring.

surgery, patient can be given a period of 1–2 years for natural conception. On the other hand, patients with pain not responding to medical management and infertility should undergo laparoscopy as early as possible. Expectant management, medical treatment, surgical treatment, and ART are available for treatment of infertility among endometriosis.

Effective, evidence-based treatments of endometriosis associated infertility include conservative surgical therapy followed by assisted reproductive technologies. Patients with infertility may not be benefited with medical therapy. Although theoretically advantageous, there is no evidence that the combination of medical and surgical treatments can significantly enhance fertility rather it may unnecessarily delay further fertility treatment.

■ EXPECTANT MANAGEMENT

Despite significantly lower fecundity rate when compared to women without endometriosis, women with mild-to-moderate endometriosis are still able to conceive in the absence of any medical or surgical intervention.[18] The option of expectant management may be reasonable for patients with mild to moderate disease where the fecundity rate is 2.4–3.0% and younger age with good ovarian reserve. Expectant management delays the start of effective treatment in those with severe disease. Patient should be counseled in detail prior to treating severe endometriosis. Invariably, they are treated as unexplained infertility and laparoscopy only can pick up. They may be advised to go to ART, which might reduce the time to achieve pregnancy.

■ MEDICAL MANAGEMENT

Although medical management is effective in relieving pain associated with endometriosis, it is ineffective in the treatment of endometriosis-associated infertility. There is no benefit from ovarian suppression, but it delays conception.[19]

Medications used as endometriosis therapy include:
- Combined oral contraceptives
- Progestins
- Danazol
- Gonadotropin-releasing hormone agonists
- Aromatase inhibitors
- Dienogest

At present, there is insufficient data to evaluate the efficacy of aromatase inhibitors, selective estrogen receptor modulators (SERMs), and progesterone antagonists in medical management of endometriosis-related infertility.

Ovarian suppression is not recommended for women who wish to conceive since there was no difference in PR or LBR following ovarian suppression versus Placebo or no treatment at all. Review of 25 trials—Meta-analysis by Hughes et al., 2007—showed no evidence to support the role of newer medical therapies in endometriosis-associated infertility (Cochrane database).[19]

■ SURGICAL MANAGEMENT

Aim of the surgical management is to regain the pelvic anatomy and remove the endometriotic deposits. Laparoscopy preferred over laparotomy and it is cost effective with minimal tissue damage and faster recovery with shorter hospital stay.

In stage I/II endometriosis, laparoscopic ablation of endometrial implants has been associated with a small but significant improvement in live birth rates. There is no evidence that the outcome is affected by the method of ablation, either electrosurgery or laser surgery. Resection or ablation for minimal or mild endometriosis: Canadian Collaborative Group [randomized controlled trial (RCT)] Marcoux et al, 1997[20] shows a positive outcome whereas study by Parazzini et al., 1999 was not significant.[21]

In infertile women with AFS/ASRM stage I/II endometriosis, clinicians should perform operative laparoscopy (excision or ablation of the endometriosis lesions) including adhesiolysis, rather than performing diagnostic laparoscopy only, to increase ongoing pregnancy rates (Evidence level A).

In infertile women with AFS/ASRM stage I/II endometriosis, clinicians may consider CO_2 laser vaporization of endometriosis, instead of monopolar electrocoagulation, since laser vaporization is associated with higher cumulative spontaneous pregnancy rates (Evidence level A).[22]

In stage III/IV endometriosis with no other identifiable infertility factors, overall data suggests that conservative surgical treatment may increase fertility.[23] In more severe stages of endometriosis, a surgical approach that normalizes pelvic anatomic distortion can enhance fertility either alone or through ART.

As per three high-quality prospective studies, crude spontaneous pregnancy rate after laparoscopic surgery is 57–69% (moderate endometriosis) 52–68% (severe endometriosis), after expectant management 33% (moderate endometriosis), and 0% (severe endometriosis) conceived.

IN VITRO FERTILIZATION: THERAPEUTIC OPTION IN STAGE III AND IV ENDOMETRIOSIS

In infertile women with endometrioma smaller than 3 cm, cystectomy prior to ART does not improve pregnancy rates.[24] (Evidence level A)—In infertile women with endometrioma larger than 3 cm, there is no evidence that cystectomy prior to ART improves pregnancy rates.[25] In women with endometrioma larger than 3 cm, (arbitrary) cystectomy is indicated prior to ART when it is associated with pain or inaccessibility of follicles (Evidence level GPP). Excision of endometrioma is strongly recommended in infertile women, when there is suspicion of malignancy or when there is potential rupture during pregnancy or torsion of the cyst.[24] However, if endometrioma resection is performed, it is critical to proceed conservatively and to minimize compromization of ovarian blood supply and preserve normal ovarian tissue **(Figs. 6A to C)**.

Laparoscopic cystectomy for ovarian endometriomas greater than 4 cm can improve fertility compared to cyst drainage and coagulation, which is also associated with a high risk of cyst recurrence.[26] Possible adverse consequence of cystectomy is the loss of viable ovarian cortex leading to decrease in ovarian reserve. Therefore, care must be taken to preserve as much ovarian tissue as possible. Hydrosalpinges reduce IVF pregnancy rates by approximately 50%, and hence salpingectomy or proximal tubal occlusion prior to ART should be done.

Postsurgical patients need more gonadotrophins and have reduced E2 levels.

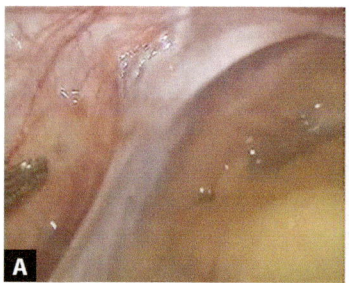 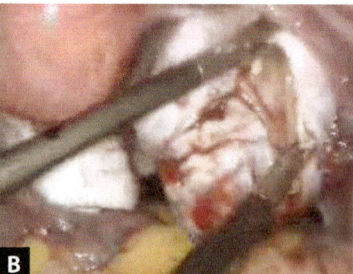 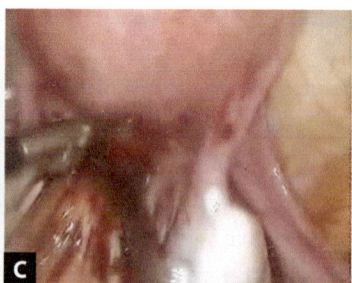

Figs. 6A to C: Superficial endometriosis, endometrioma, and deep infiltrating endometriosis.

Decrease in oocyte number, but no difference in implantation rate, pregnancy rate, or miscarriage rate.

In infertile women with ovarian endometrioma undergoing surgery, clinicians should perform excision of the endometrioma capsule, instead of drainage and electrocoagulation of the endometrioma wall, to increase spontaneous pregnancy rates (Evidence level A).

The Guideline Development Group (GDG) recommends that clinicians should counsel women with endometrioma regarding the risks of reduced ovarian function after surgery and the possible loss of the ovary. The decision to proceed with surgery should be considered carefully if the woman has had previous ovarian surgery (Evidence level GPP).

In infertile women with AFS/ASRM stage III/IV endometriosis, instead of expectant management, one can consider operative laparoscopy, to increase spontaneous pregnancy rates (Evidence level B).

Cochrane review: Three RCTs analyzed excision of endometrioma. Meta-analysis of 597 patients 13 out of 24 were analyzed, decrease in AFC postoperatively, 9 studies out of 11 decreases in anti-Müllerian hormone (AMH). Risk vs. benefit should be counseled. USG-directed cyst aspiration is associated with mixed results. There is an increased incidence of infection.

Surgery prior to treatment with ART in women with deep infiltrative endometriosis (DIE): There is no evidence to recommend performing surgical excision of DIE prior to ART in infertile women with endometriosis, to improve reproductive outcomes. However, these women often suffer from pain, requiring surgical treatment.

The effectiveness of surgical excision of deep nodular lesions before treatment with ART is not well established with regard to reproductive outcome (Evidence level C).

Cochrane meta-analysis of laparoscopic salpingectomy or proximal tubal occlusion has better conception rates in patients with hydrosalpinx.

Repeat surgery only rarely increases the fecundability and these patients may be better treated through ART. In patients with repeated IVF failure, surgery can be advised which can improve the spontaneous or ART conception (Littmann et al.).

COMBINATION OF MEDICAL AND SURGICAL THERAPY

There is no evidence to show that combination of medical and surgical therapy significantly enhances fertility. Moreover, it may unnecessarily delay further fertility therapy. There are certain conditions such as associated adenomyosis, where two to three doses of GnRh agonists prior to frozen embryo transfer (FET), may improve the pregnancy rates through ART.

SUPEROVULATION AND INTRAUTERINE INSEMINATION

The ASRM guidelines suggest that superovulation (SO)/IUI may be a viable treatment option for women who had surgical diagnosis and treatment for stage I or II endometriosis as an alternative to IVF.[27] SO/IUI depends upon the age, duration of infertility, stage of the disease and done within 6 months of surgery. Treatment with IUI improves fertility in minimal to mild endometriosis. (RCOG guideline October 2006). Gonadotropins + IUI significantly improve the results as compared with no treatment (26% vs. 8%; RR

3.3; 95% CI 1.2–9.4). Role of IUI without COH is uncertain (Evidence Level B).

Single sitting after 36 hours of trigger is ideal and double sitting IUI may be recommended for poor male factor. In infertile women stage I/II endometriosis, clinicians may perform IUI with COS instead of expectant management, as it increases live birth rates (Evidence level C). Clinicians may perform IUI with COS, instead of IUI alone, as it increases pregnancy rates (Evidence level C). IUI with COS should be done within 6 months after surgical treatment, since pregnancy rates are similar to those achieved in unexplained infertility (Evidence level C). There is increased risk of recurrence seen with IUI when compared to IVF because of spontaneous ovulation (which is a risk factor for endometrioma).

INDICATIONS FOR ASSISTED REPRODUCTIVE TECHNOLOGY

- Associated tubal factor
- Male infertility
- Failed IUI in minimal-to-mild endometriosis
- Failed IUI in moderate-to-severe endometriosis of < 35 years
- Moderate to severe endometriosis of beyond 35 years
- Diminished ovarian reserve
- Prior surgical treatment
- EFI score is <4
- Failed natural/ovulation conception over a period of 2 years when EFI score is beyond 4.

While endometriosis may affect IVF results compared to male and tubal factor infertility, IVF is likely to maximize the cycle fecundity for those with endometriosis, especially in those with distortion of pelvic anatomy due to moderate or severe disease when compared to expectant or surgical management.

There is currently insufficient data to clarify whether ovarian endometrioma should be removed prior to IVF, as there are chances of reduction in ovarian reserve. If all healthy growing follicles can be reached without damaging the endometrioma during COS, even a cyst over 4 cm does not require surgery in asymptomatic patients. Even smaller cysts which interfere with oocyte pick up has to removed surgically. Accidental puncture of endometrioma during oocyte pick up, clinician should give antibiotics and postpone the embryo transfer. Patients having pain and suspicious of malignant change in endometrioma should undergo surgery.

Clinicians can prescribe GnRh agonists for a period of 3–6 months prior to treatment with assisted reproductive technologies to improve clinical pregnancy rates in infertile women with endometriosis.[28]

CONCLUSION

Ultimately, the optimal method for treatment of endometriosis-associated infertility must be individualized, based on patient's parameters. Many factors must be taken into account including distorted pelvic anatomy, ovarian reserve, male factor, age, presence of endometriomas, and duration of infertility. Depending upon the patient, current treatment options may include expectant management, surgery with or without ovulation induction/IUI or IVF.

REFERENCES

1. Coomarasamy A, Shafi M, Davila GW, Chan KK. Gynecologic and obstetric surgery: challenges and management options. USA: John Wiley & Sons; 2016.
2. FOGSI Endometriosis Committee 2014-2016. (2016). Good clinical practice recommendations on endometriosis. [online] Available from: https://www.fogsi.org/

wp-content/uploads/2017/01/GCRP-2017-final.pdf. [Last accessed June, 2023].
3. Ballweg ML. Big picture of endometriosis helps provide guidance on approach to teens: comparative historical data show endo starting younger, is more severe. J Pediatr Adolesc Gynecol. 2003; 16(3):S21-6.
4. Child TJ, Tan SL. Endometriosis. Drugs. 2001; 61(12):1735-50.
5. Cramer DW, Missmer SA. The epidemiology of endometriosis. Ann N Y Acad Sci. 2002; 955(1):11-22.
6. Bendigeri T, Ghuge A, Bhusane K, Begum S, Warty N, Sawant R, et al. Stage-wise comparison of anti-endometrial-antibodies against peptides of SLP2, TMOD3 and TPM3 in diagnosis of endometriosis. Fertil Steril. 2015;104(3):e162.
7. Chapron C, Marcellin L, Borghese B, Santulli P. Rethinking mechanisms, diagnosis, and management of endometriosis. Nat Rev Endocrinol. 2019;15(11):666-82.
8. Leyland N, Casper R, Laberge P, Singh SS, Allen L, Arendas K, et al. Endometriosis: diagnosis and management. J Endometr. 2010;2(3):107-34.
9. American College of Obstetricians and Gynecologists. Practice bulletin no. 114: management of endometriosis. Obstet Gynecol. 2010;116(1):223-36.
10. Johnson NP, Hummelshoj L, World Endometriosis Society Montpellier Consortium, Abrao MS, Adamson GD, Allaire C, et al. Consensus on current management of endometriosis. Hum Reprod. 2013;28(6):1552-68.
11. Dunselman GA, Vermeulen N, Becker C, Calhaz-Jorge C, D'Hooghe T, De Bie B, et al. ESHRE guideline: management of women with endometriosis. Hum Reprod. 2014;29(3):400-12.
12. Bulletti C, Coccia ME, Battistoni S, Borini A. Endometriosis and infertility. Journal of Assisted Reproduction and Genetics. 2010;27:441-7.
13. Hudson QJ, Perricos A, Wenzl R, Yotova I. Challenges in uncovering non-invasive biomarkers of endometriosis. Experimental Biology and Medicine. 2020;245(5):437-47.
14. Vercellini P, Viganò P, Somigliana E, Fedele L. Endometriosis: pathogenesis and treatment. Nature Reviews Endocrinology. 2014;10(5):261-75.
15. Verkauf BS. Incidence, symptoms, and signs of endometriosis in fertile and infertile women. J Fla Med Assoc. 1987;74(9):671-5.
16. Pellicer A, Navarro J, Bosch E, Garrido N, Garcia-Velasco JA, Remohí J, et al. Endometrial quality in infertile women with endometriosis. Ann N Y Acad Sci. 2001; 943(1):122-30.
17. Cook AS, Adamson GD. The role of the endometriosis fertility index (EFI) and endometriosis scoring systems in predicting infertility outcomes. Curr Obstet Gynecol. 2013;2(3):186-94.
18. Eleftheriou G, Butera R, Manzo L. Holoprosencephaly in clomiphene-induced pregnancy: a possible association? A case report and literature review. Clin Exp Obstet Gynecol. 2012;39(4):1256.
19. Hughes E, Brown J, Collins JJ, Farquhar C, Fedorkow DM, Vanderkerchove P. Ovulation suppression for endometriosis for women with subfertility. Cochrane Database Syst Rev. 2007(3):CD000155.
20. Marcoux S, Maheux R, Bérubé S, Canadian Collaborative Group on Endometriosis. Laparoscopic surgery in infertile women with minimal or mild endometriosis. N Engl J Med. 1997;337(4):217-22.
21. Parazzini F. Ablation of lesions or no treatment in minimal-mild endometriosis in infertile women: a randomized trial. Gruppo Italiano per lo Studio dell'Endometriosi. Hum Reprod. 1999;14(5):1332-4.
22. Dunselman GA, Vermeulen N, Becker C, Calhaz-Jorge C, D'Hooghe T, De Bie B, et al. ESHRE guideline: management of women with endometriosis. Hum Reprod. 2014;29(3):400-12.
23. Schenken RS. Modern concepts of endometriosis. Classification and its consequences for therapy. J Reprod Med. 1998;43 (3 Suppl):269-75.
24. Garcia-Velasco JA, Mahutte NG, Corona J, Zúñiga V, Gilés J, Arici A, et al. Removal of

endometriomas before in vitro fertilization does not improve fertility outcomes: a matched, case-control study. Fertil Steril. 2004;81(5):1194-7.
25. Benschop L, Farquhar C, van der Poel N, Heineman MJ. Interventions for women with endometrioma prior to assisted reproductive technology. Cochrane Database Syst Rev. 2010(11):CD008571.
26. Chapron C, Vercellini P, Barakat H, Vieira M, Dubuisson JB. Management of ovarian endometriomas. Hum Reprod Update. 2002; 8(6):591-7.
27. Zeng C, Xu JN, Zhou Y, Zhou YF, Zhu SN, Xue Q. Reproductive performance after surgery for endometriosis: predictive value of the revised American Fertility Society classification and the endometriosis fertility index. Gynecol Obstet Invest. 2014;77(3): 180-5.
28. Schleedoorn MJ, Nelen WL, Dunselman GA, Vermeulen N, EndoKey Group, Andersson EA, et al. Selection of key recommendations for the management of women with endometriosis by an international panel of patients and professionals. Hum Reprod. 2016;31(6):1208-18.

CHAPTER 9

Future and Stem Cell Therapy

Kalyan B Barmade, Manisha K Barmade, Anand B Barmade

■ INTRODUCTION

The human endometrium undergoes cycles of growth and regression with each menstrual cycle. Adult progenitor stem cells may cause this. Progenitor stem cells have an enhanced capacity to generate endometriosis if shed in a retrograde fashion. These cells reside in the uterus. Mesenchymal stem cells can also be involved in the pathogenesis of endometriosis.

■ STEM CELLS WITHIN THE UTERUS

The human uterine endometrium consists of glandular epithelium and stroma that are completely renewed in each monthly menstrual cycle. Cyclic endometrial renewal depends on a small pool of tissue-specific multipotential stem cells.[1,2]

Under cyclic hormonal changes, stem cells migrate and give rise to progenitor cells that create specific types of differentiated cells, e.g., epithelial, stromal, and vascular cells. These endogenous stem cells allow the rapid regeneration of the endometrium necessary to support pregnancy.[3]

There is new school of thought that endometrial regeneration arises from bone marrow-derived cells.

■ STEM CELLS IN ENDOMETRIOSIS

In the menstrual blood, progenitor cells are found, which can give hypothesis that it would be responsible for endometriosis.

Epithelial cells in a few endometriosis lesions are monoclonal, suggesting a single cell origin, possibly by an endometrial stem/progenitor cell.

Leyendecker et al. showed that significantly more basalis layer was shed in the menstrual flow suggesting an increased number of stem cells in this layer that can result in a propensity for endometriosis.[4]

Stemness-related genes, such as the transcription pluripotency factors *SOX2* (sex-determining region Y-box 2), *NANOG* (Nanog homeobox), and *OCT4* (octamer-binding protein 4) in the endometrium of reproductive-age women with and without ovarian endometriosis, have role in the regulation of self-renewal and pluripotency in embryonic stem cells and primordial germ cells.

The $CD146^+CD140b^+$ population is located at the perivascular region in both functional and basal layers and can differentiate into osteogenic, myogenic, adipogenic, and chondrogenic lineages, as well as fibroblasts and smooth muscle cells.[5]

Menstrual stem cells (MenSCs) were first identified from menstrual blood in 2007, which can effectively propagate for over 68 population doublings with normal karyotype. MenSCs express markers, namely CD29, CD9, CD13, CD44, CD41a, CD73, CD59, CD90, and CD105 but not CD19, CD34, CD45, CD117, CD130, or HLA-DR.[6]

Endometriosis alters the peritoneal microenvironment of women, in which the immune response, angiogenesis, cell proliferation, cell adhesion, and apoptosis are uniquely regulated in peritoneal fluid (PF). A specific protein expression pattern is present in PF with deep infiltrating endometriosis (DIE) compared in PF with non-DIE.[7]

STEM CELL-TARGETED THERAPIES

Current treatments rely on the manipulation of a woman's menstrual cycle to prevent the establishment and growth of lesions by suppressing ovarian function and inducing a hypoestrogenic state. Hormonal contraceptives are not suitable for everyone and can have off-target effects. It is becoming increasingly pertinent that new endometriosis therapies must target lesion establishment and lesion progression because both may occur with every menstrual cycle.

Stem cells are undifferentiated cells that have the ability to self-renew as well as to produce more differentiated daughter cells. Broadly, stem cells can be divided into two categories: embryonic and adult. Embryonic stem cells are derived from blastocysts. Adult stem cells, derived from postembryonic cell lineages, have been described in a number of different organ systems and have been best characterized in the hematopoietic system.

While stem/progenitor cells' presence in menstrual debris is likely to play a crucial role in the survival of a menstrual fragment and then its formation of a lesion.

- *Sorafenib* is a protein tyrosine kinase inhibitor targeting RAF kinases, growth factor receptors including c-KIT, and PDGFRB, eSF and eMSC markers. As a potent inhibitor of angiogenesis.
- *Cabergoline:* In direct coculture of eutopic or ectopic eMSCs with human umbilical vein endothelial cells (HUVECs), a subset of eMSCs differentiated into CD31þ endothelial-like cells and contributed to the formation of tube-like structure. Cabergoline, a dopamine receptor 2 agonist, partly inhibited CD31 marker expression on eMSCs but did not inhibit eMSC incorporation into tube structure.
- *Statins* have also been investigated for their antiangiogenic properties. Lipid-soluble statins (simvastatin, lovastatin, and atorvastatin) were effective in inhibition of growth and invasiveness of human endometrial stromal (HES) cells in invitro studies. These findings may have clinical relevance in treatment of endometriosis.

While endometrial stem/progenitor cells are promising therapeutic targets for endometriosis, more research focused on the perivascular or clonogenic eMSC population, rather than heterogeneous endometrial cell cultures, is required. Targeting endometrial stem/progenitor cells will require care, as these drugs will also affect endometrial growth, which will adversely affect women desiring pregnancy. The effects of blocking angiogenesis on fertility and pregnancy also need investigation.

REFERENCES

1. Maruyama T, Masuda H, Ono M, Kajitani T, Yoshimura Y. Human uterine stem/progenitor cells: Their possible role in uterine physiology and pathology. Reproduction. 2010;140:11-22.
2. Padykula HA. Regeneration in the primate uterus. In: Wynn RM, Jollie WP (Eds). Biology of the uterus. New Delhi: Springer; 1989. pp. 279-88
3. Chan RW, Schwab KE, Gargett CE. Clonogenicity of human endometrial epithelial and stromal cells. Biol Reprod. 2004;70:1738-50.

4. Leyendecker G, Herbertz M, Kunz G, Mall G. Endometriosis results from the dislocation of basal endometrium. Hum Reprod. 2002; 17: 2725-36.
5. Masuda H, Anwar SS, Buhring HJ, Rao JR, Gargett CE. A novel marker of human endometrial mesenchymal stem-like cells. Cell Transplant. 2012;21(10):2201-14.
6. Meng X, Ichim TE, Zhong J, Rogers A, Yin Z, Jackson J, et al. Endometrial regenerative cells: a novel stem cell population. J Transl Med. 2007;5:57.
7. Perricos A, Wenzl R, Husslein H, Eiwegger T, Gstoettner M, Weinhaeusel A, et al. Does the use of the "Proseek® multiplex oncology I panel" on peritoneal fluid allow a better insight in the pathophysiology of endometriosis, and in particular deep-infiltrating endometriosis? J Clin Med. 2020; 9:2009.

CHAPTER 10

Endometriosis and Intrauterine Insemination Protocols

Rohan Palshetkar, Manisha Nandi

■ BACKGROUND

Assisted reproduction technology (ART) is often used as the first-line treatment in infertile women with endometriosis. The American Society for Reproductive Medicine and the European Society of Human Reproduction and Embryology (ESHRE) guidelines recommend intrauterine insemination (IUI) in women with minimal-to-mild endometriosis.[1]

MILD OR MINIMAL ENDOMETRIOSIS AND INFERTILITY

The mechanisms underlying reproductive failure are subtle and still remain controversial, especially in patients with endometriosis, the adverse effects on reproduction may be observed due to the following:

- Toxic effects primarily affecting the quality of the gametes and embryos, with impaired tubal motility: as the endometriotic implants predominantly release the proinflammatory cytokines [interleukin-1β,6,8, and tumor necrosis factor alpha (TNF α)], hormones play a role too as progesterone and estradiol tend to attract macrophages and promote the release of vascular endothelial growth factor (VEGF), and interleukin-8, which creates a state of chronic inflammation and furthermore causes impairment of fertility in patients with endometriosis.
- An altered and hostile follicular environment with high proinflammatory cytokines
- An increase in apoptosis of the granulosa cells
- The peritoneal macrophages cause enhanced phagocytosis of the sperms
- Reduction in the rate of fertilization for women undergoing ART
- Impaired implantation and poor endometrial response due to chronic inflammatory changes and an overt response to the endometrial antigens by increase in the production of antibodies

Minimal/mild endometriosis usually alters the outcome of controlled ovarian hyperstimulation (COH) in IUI with up to 30% drop the rate of clinical pregnancy **(Fig. 1)**. Recently, two randomized controlled trials (RCTs) have supported that COH–IUI is considered to be more beneficial than opting for no treatment for patients with pelvic endometriosis. Tummon and colleagues in their study stated that overall live births was increased by fivefold after treatment with COH–IUI.[2]

MODERATE AND SEVERE ENDOMETRIOSIS: IMPACT ON REPRODUCTION

Along with the previously stated factors, the following plays a role in moderate-to-severe disease:

- Impaired release of oocytes due to ovarian endometriomas and adhesions

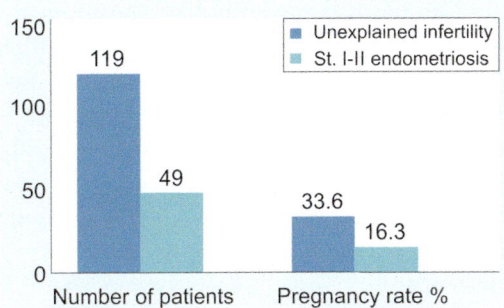

Fig. 1: Outcome of patients with unexplained infertility and mild to moderate endometriosis.

- Impaired tubal motility
- Lack of sperm migration due to blockage

Van der Houwen et al. in their study reported that IUI is a valuable treatment option for subfertility management in patients with severe form of the disease, i.e., moderate-to-severe stages of endometriosis. The pregnancy rates of 29% in women with severe endometriosis after 6 cycles of IUI were noted. In another recent study, the clinical pregnancy rates in women with ovarian endometriomas were found to be low as compared to patients with unexplained infertility (14.3% vs. 28.9%; p value = 0.10). There was a trend in the favor of unexplained infertility, but the number was found to be probably too low to enable researchers to observe the statistically significance of the differences that were found from this aspect. It has also been noted that the majority of the couples in the study had received no more than four cycles of IUI treatment. Although this also reflects upon the daily practice, as we cannot overall exclude that there is a possibility of more number of cycles of IUI could have ensured a significantly higher difference in clinical pregnancy rate in the study groups.

■ CONSIDERATION ON PROTOCOLS

In subfertile patients with minimal-to-mild endometriosis, IUI with the administration of gonadotropins and controlled ovarian stimulation (COS) could be useful, other than preferring no treatment and IUI only as it has been found to increase respectively, 5.7 and 5.2 times the clinical pregnancy rates. The National Institute for Health and Care Excellence (NICE) guidelines current recommendation states that IUI is to be used to treat minimal-to-mild endometriosis after counseling the couples that ovarian stimulation might increase the clinical pregnancy rates when compared to opting for expectant management; however, the benefits of offering an unstimulated IUI is unclear (NICE : Grade A recommendation).

Alternatively, many clinicians might opt for IUI cycles with COH following 6 months of surgery, as the clinical pregnancy rates are observed to be similar to that achieved for patients with unexplained subfertility.

A recent Cochrane review has reported that no statistically significant difference has been noted between the different timing protocols applied for IUI, which includes the administration of human chorionic gonadotropin (hCG) (recombinant or urinary), and detecting the luteinizing hormone (LH)s surge with the subsequent use of gonadotropin-releasing hormone agonist (GnRHa). Moreover, owing to limited evidences at present, there are no recommendations that specify the techniques of semen sample preparation. As for the normal samples, it is not clear yet as to whether there are any advantages in relation to the isolation and use of the most motile spermatozoa before insemination or if results obtained might be similar with the usage of the whole population of spermatozoa in the sample.

Letrozole vs. Clomiphene Citrate

From the year 2007 to 2010, 433 cycles were included in 136 patients in an intention-to-treat analysis (A total of 220 IUI cycles in 69 patients for the IUI with Letrozole group vs. 213 cycles in 67 patients in the IUI with Clomiphene Citrate group). The study results found no statistically significant differences between the groups with regards to the age of the patients, duration of infertility, basal body mass index, and basal hormonal levels (Prolactin, estradiol, FSH, and LH), the percentage of patients with stage I/II endometriosis or with the time period from surgery and commencement of first IUI cycle **(Table 1)**. **Flowchart 1** depicts the events and allocation of patients in the study. Six and five participants in letrozole and Clomiphene group, respectively, dropped out from the study after negative reports of serum beta-hCG level with three cycles of IUI and they opted for in vitro fertilization (IVF). With 125 patients (422 cycles) who decided to remain for the protocol analysis.

The clinical reproductive results of the study are given in **Table 2**. The number of follicles >18 mm during the COS was statistically found to be significant (higher in the Clomiphene group) (2.90 ± 0.40 vs. 1.40 ± 0.20). No significant statistical difference was found to be of no significance with regards to the pretreatment thickness of the endometrium (ET) between the two study groups. Further, an increase in the endometrial thickness on the day of hCG injection was noted in the Letrozole group (8.80 ± 1.20 vs. 8.20 ± 0.90 mm). The serum estradiol level on the day of hCG injection was significantly higher in the Clomiphene group. Moreover, no difference was noted between the two study groups in terms of duration of COS, i.e., average hCG day and progesterone level. No statistically significant difference was noted with regards to clinical pregnancy rate/cycle as per the applied protocol or in intention-to-treat analyses (16.30 vs. 14.90%; 15.9 vs. 14% in women treated with letrozole and Clomiphene, respectively). They also noted no differences in the pregnancy rate/

TABLE 1: Comparison of the group characteristics; pregnancy and abortion rates amongst the different stimulation protocols.

	CC + FSH	HMG + FSH	L + FSH + HMG	CC + FSH after Leupride depot
Age (y)*	32.4 ± 3.9	33.5 ± 3.9	32.8 ± 3.5	33.8 ± 3.8
Duration of infertility (y)*	3.0 ± 1.9	3.4 ± 1.8	3.3 ± 2.3	3.6 ± 2.4
Primary infertility	75	33	169	44
Secondary infertility	56	26	103	28
Pregnancy rate	18/131	11/59	61/272	26/72
	(13.7%)[†]	(18.6%)[†]	(22.4%)[†]t	(36.1%)[†]
Abortion rate	4/18	2/11	10/61	4/26
Ectopic rate	(22.2%) 1/61 (1.6%)	(18.2%)	(16.4%)	(15.4%)

*Values are means ± SD.
[†]$p < 0.05$
(cc: clomiphene citrate; FSH: follicle-stimulating hormone; HMG: human menopausal gonadotropin)

Endometriosis and Intrauterine Insemination Protocols

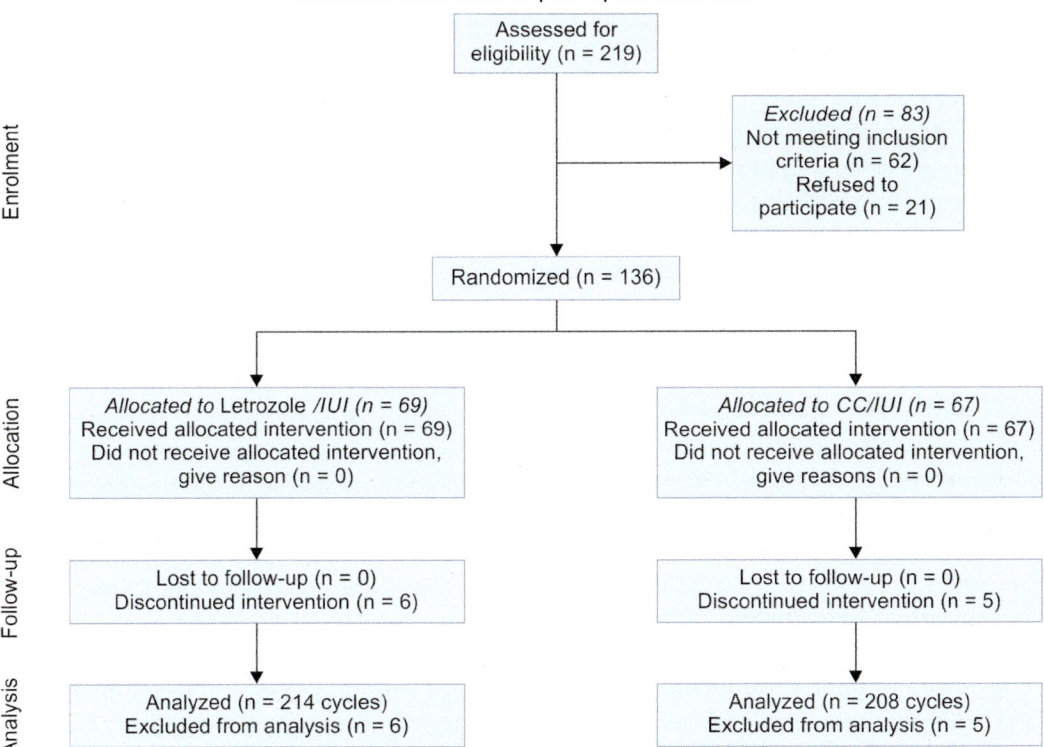

Flowchart 1: Events and participant allocation.

(CC: clomiphene citrate; IUI: intrauterine insemination)

TABLE 2: Presents the participant database and a comparison of the two groups (Letrozole vs. Clomiphene Citrate).

	Group A (letrozole/IUI) (n = 69)	%	Group B (CC/IUI) (n = 67)	%	p-value
Age (years)	31.3 ± 2.2		30.7 ± 2.7		0.12
Duration of infertility (years)	2.8 ± 0.7		2.7 ± 0.8		0.33
BMI (kg/m^2)	24.7 ± 2.9		25.4 ± 2.3		0.52
Clinical presentation					
Minimal endometriosis	63	91.3	59	88	0.86
Mild endometriosis	6	8.7	8	12	0.32
Time interval laparoscopy/first IUI cycle (years)	0.83 ± 0.11		0.79 ± 0.24		0.18
Day 3 FSH (IU/mL)	7.1 ± 1.6		6.8 ± 1.4		0.16
Day 3 LH (IU/mL)	5.4 ± 1.8		5.2 ± 1.7		0.14
Day 3 E2 (pg/mL)	48.4 ± 10.8		43.7 ± 11.4		0.43

(CC: clomiphene citrate; E2: estradiol; FSH: follicle-stimulating hormone; IUI: intrauterine insemination; LH: luteinizing hormone)

patient (50.70 vs. 46.30% in Letrozole and Clomiphene group of patients, respectively).

No significant difference in terms of clinical pregnancy rates after four cycles of IUI (67.90 vs. 58.90% in the Letrozole and Clomiphene group of patients, respectively). After application of the intention-to-treat analysis, clinical pregnancy rate after four cycles was 64.7% in the letrozole group and was 57% in the Clomiphene group, which was statistically found to be nonsignificant.[3]

However, Jee et al. and coworkers have stated that the aromatase inhibitors (Letrozole) are rapidly eliminated from body owing to the drug's short half-life (approximately 50 hours) as compared to a longer half-life of Clomiphene Citrate Zu-isomer (>1 month). The supraphysiologic concentrations of estrogen can happen with the use of Clomiphene without a central suppression of follicle-stimulating hormone (FSH); because normal estrogen receptor-mediated feedback mechanism gets blocked, which results in the growth of multiple follicles and results in higher rates of multiple pregnancies when compared to letrozole-stimulated cycles. Hence, when we need multiple mature follicles to develop, letrozole alone may not be the best choice for COS to occur. Mitwally and Casper in their study reported that in patients stimulated with Letrozole had a much thicker endometrium as when compared with clomiphene citrate. This may be due to the improvement of vascularization as observed in recent Doppler studies.

Superovulation with letrozole has been found to be not more effective as compared to clomiphene alone when used in an IUI cycle for patients with mild endometriosis who had failed pregnancy following 6–12 months from the date of laparoscopy. As it is a cheaper option, clomiphene could be considered to be the reasonable drug of choice as an oral drug with regards to costeffectiveness.[3]

Clomiphene Citrate/Human Menopausal Gonadotropin

A retrospective study has recently evaluated the different COH protocols [human menopausal gonadotropin (HMG) FSH; Clomiphene/FSH; HMG/FSH after GnRH agonist treatment protocols; Clomiphene/FSH after GnRH agonist] for IUI cycles in women with mild endometriosis and infertility. They had included a total of 393 patients with laparoscopic diagnosis of stage I/II endometriosis in accordance to the rAFS classification. In total, 534 IUI cycles with different COH protocols were then conducted. 131 cycles of CC and gonadotropin (CC/FSH) stimulation, 59 stimulated cycles with only gonadotropin (HMG FSH), 272 COH cycles with gonadotropin immediately after GnRH agonist and a total of 72 cycles of clomiphene and gonadotropin after GnRH agonist treatment. It was noted that after GnRHa protocol, the researchers preferred to use gonadotropins alone as the COS protocol, as the first cycle of COS. When the first cycle had a failure to achieve pregnancy, then clomiphene with gonadotropin (Clomiphene, FSH) was used for the second cycle. The primary outcome of analysis was pregnancy rate, which was then defined as levels of serum beta-hCG more than 5 mIU/mL on the 16th day after performing the IUI cycle.

The COH protocols after treatment with GnRH agonists had reported a highly significant cycle fecundity compared to the protocols without the use of GnRH agonists in patients with minimal/mild endometriosis. Furthermore, the protocol of Clomiphene and FSH after GnRHa treatment had revealed as to be the most effective hyperstimulation protocol, for IUI in patients with Stage I/II endometriosis. On the basis of their finding, it was suggested that treatment with GnRH agonists and the superovulation is very much necessary for infertility patients with pelvic endometriosis.[4]

Werbrouck et al. and colleagues had observed a pregnancy rate of 20% per cycle; their study was retrospective and had included use of hMG in most of the cycles (116 of 137) 6-12 months after surgery. Tiitinen and Isaksson in a retrospective study had included Clomiphene/hMG for COH for the participants; however, IUI was done in 130 of the 233 cycles. Timed intercourse after direct intraperitoneal insemination was done for the other cycles.[5]

Dmowski et al. had reported in their study that if superovulation and IUI is to be performed in patients with endometriosis, a maximum of three to four cycles should be allowed. Although, there is no current guidelines with regards to the best protocol that can be used in patients with endometriosis undergoing IUI cycles.

The use of gonadotropins in the stimulated protocols mostly have a significantly high risk of ovarian hyperstimulation syndrome (OHSS) and of a higher risk of multiple pregnancies. In a Cochrane review, meta-analysis of six studies including 456 patients with history of unexplained subfertility, with mild male factor in the males and endometriosis in the female partners, observed a difference of 5.7% in the pregnancy rate with gonadotropins in the IUI cycles as compared with Clomiphene/IUI cycles; this difference was, however, not found to be statistically significant (95% CI: 1.0, 12.5).[6]

The rationale for COS in patients with endometriomas has always been to study and treat the disorders the endocrine and ovulation, which includes luteinized unruptured follicle syndrome, premature LH surges, and abnormal follicular growth. Moreover, COS can cause some concerns in women with endometriosis and hence should be strictly considered based on the individual patient profile.

INTRAUTERINE INSEMINATION: CLINICAL IMPACT

The optimum number of attempts with IUI cycles has always been a challenge and a question while counseling the patients. One recent study has reported that IUI cycles for patients with unexplained infertility/endometriosis should be for three cycles and not more.

However, the debate of the present scenario is whether IUI cycles with COH is better when compared to unstimulated cycle of IUI. A RCT conducted recently has failed to report an advantage of stimulated over the unstimulated cycles in patients with endometriosis. However, a Cochrane review has supported Clomiphene Citrate and suggested that it has a positive role when used for women with endometriosis. Another recent study has observed an increase in the clinical pregnancy rate in women treated with stimulated cycles of IUI allowing a maximum of six cycles as compared to three IUI cycles without COS followed by up to three IUI cycles with COS which has supported the Cochrane review.

CONCLUSION

A significant number of patients seek ART for a successful pregnancy, especially those with poor ovarian reserve or other identified factors causing infertility. Studies have found that for infertile women with only endometriosis (i.e., patency of fallopian tubes and normal ovarian reserve), IUI treatment is an effective treatment that can be offered for infertility due to endometriosis. The optimal treatment plan often provides to be a topic of clinical debates and there exists little to no evidence to provide clinicians with robust guidance at present. A sequence of IUI cycles in women with endometriosis is considered to be a less expensive and aggressive approach than opting for IVF. Hence, IUI cycles should be offered as a viable and a valuable approach for achieving a successful pregnancy.

REFERENCES

1. Cai H, Xie J, Shi J, Wang H. Efficacy of intrauterine insemination in women with endometrioma-associated subfertility: analysis using propensity score matching. BMC Pregnancy Childbirth. 2022;22:12.
2. Fadhlaoui A, Bouquet de la Jolinière J, Feki A. Endometriosis and Infertility: How and When to Treat? Front Surg. 2014;1:24.
3. Abu Hashim H, El Rakhawy M, Abd Elaal I. Randomized comparison of superovulation with letrozole vs. clomiphene citrate in an IUI program for women with recently surgically treated minimal to mild endometriosis. Acta Obstet Gynecol Scand. 2012;91(3):338-45.
4. Wang RS, Yang PS, Au HK, Sheen TC, Tzeng CR. Hyperstimulation protocol for IUI in the treatment of infertility associated with minimal or mild endometriosis. Fertil Steril. 2002;77:S27.
5. Werbrouck E, Spiessens C, Meuleman C, D'Hooghe T. No difference in cycle pregnancy rate and in cumulative live-birth rate between women with surgically treated minimal to mild endometriosis and women with unexplained infertility after controlled ovarian hyperstimulation and intrauterine insemination. Fertil Steril. 2006;86(3):566-71.
6. Dmowski WP, Pry M, Ding J, Rana N. Cycle-specific and cumulative fecundity in patients with endometriosis who are undergoing controlled ovarian hyperstimulation-intrauterine insemination or in vitro fertilization-embryo transfer. Fertil Steril. 2002;78(4):750-6.

CHAPTER 11

Endometriosis and In Vitro Fertilization

Rohan Palshetkar, Mayuri More, Manisha Nandi

INTRODUCTION

Pelvic endometriosis affects 2–10% of women in the general population and accounts for 20–50% of patients who are investigated for subinfertility. Despite various extensive studies, the exact mechanisms by which endometriosis causes subfertility is not clearly understood. The in vitro fertilization and embryo transfer (IVF-ET) has become the most common method to help patients with endometriosis-associated infertility; with the use of IVF-ET, it has become possible to bypass the suspected pathology/disturbed functions, which usually affect the natural cycles by endometriosis such as alteration of folliculogenesis, ovulatory dysfunction, impaired oocyte maturation, cleavage of embryo, and implantation-related abnormalities.[1]

PELVIC ENDOMETRIOSIS AND DETERMINATION OF OOCYTE QUALITY BASED ON BIOLOGICAL MARKERS

Owing to the present ethical issues, the oocyte quality has frequently been indirectly studied, after evaluating the cumulus cells which surround the oocytes and the content of the follicular fluid. Nevertheless, these observations that usually reflect upon the competence and the quality of the inherent oocytes are yet to be explained at large.

IMPACT OF DYSREGULATED STEROIDOGENESIS

Steroidogenesis is a two-cell process, which is aided by the granulosa cell-derived paracrine factors, which promote the activity of P450 aromatase—the key enzyme for production of estrogen—and it allows for adequate aromatizable androgen synthesis for the appropriate 17-beta-estradiol production. Estradiol (E2) plays a vital role in the growth of follicles and to produce a capable oocyte that is able to accomplish the stage of maturation [Metaphase II (MII) stage] and can undergo fertilization. The deleterious effects of pelvic endometriosis on the typical physiology of the granulosa cells have been broadly described in the recent times including the changes that occur in the cell cycle, the role of increased apoptosis, and the mechanism of dysregulated molecular pathways that is involved in the growth and development of the granulosa cells. Earlier research in this field has shown that the ovarian endometriomas/endometriosis at other sites in the pelvis might have a detrimental effect on the granulosa cell steroidogenesis by P450 aromatase expression reduction **(Fig. 1)**.

Earlier studies have shown that in patients with endometriosis, there is an impairment in the mechanism of steroidogenesis, which may cause an imbalance in estrogen production: lower serum E2 levels, at the preovulatory

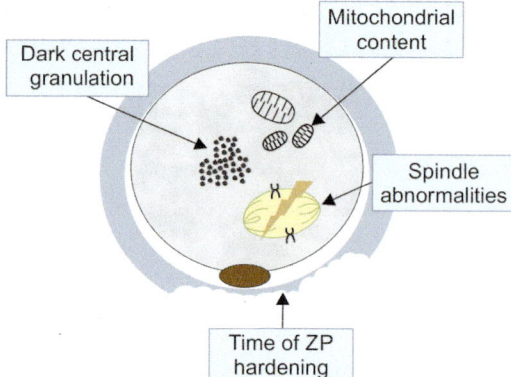

Fig. 1: Changes noted morphologically in the oocytes from patients with endometriosis. (ZP: zona pellucida)

stage, and also during luteinizing hormone (LH) surge. Also to note that following assisted reproductive technology (ART), patients with endometriosis tend to have a lower E2 concentration on the human chorionic gonadotropin (hCG) trigger day in comparison with patients without the disease.

Mechanism of Disruption of the Intrafollicular Environment

Various studies have been recently published describing how endometriosis alters the various factors presented in the follicular fluid (FF). The stages of the disease based upon the revised classification as established by the American Society for Reproductive Medicine (ASRM) has a strong importance with regards to this context.

In the recent years, concerns whether endometriosis could be the reason that modifies the status of follicular oxidative stress have been raised. It is solely based on the fact that oxidative stress acts as one of the potential factors that is in relation to the pathophysiological process of the disease, and ROS (reactive oxygen species) also promotes the chromosomal instability and meiotic abnormalities, therefore, leads to the reduction in the quality of exposed oocytes. Naturally, the oocyte gets arrested in the prophase I stage, wherein the microtubule network is found to be in a form of pseudointerphasic.

Da Broi and coworkers in their study found an elevation in the follicular concentration of 8-hydroxy-2′-deoxyguanosine, which is one of the indicators of DNA damage, has been found in the FF of patients with both mild and severe stages of the disease. Amongst the others, BDNF (brain-derived neurotrophic factor) recently has shown to have a molecular link between folliculogenesis and protection from factors contributing to oxidative stress. The unique polymorphisms noted in *BDNF* gene is closely associated with the higher incidence of the disease-related infertility with $p < 0.05$. Also in support of the fact that a unique genotype might be responsible for infertility related to the disease development, reduction in the FF BDNF concentrations ($p < 0.01$), lesser number of mature oocytes obtained ($p < 0.01$) and decrease in the rate of fertilization ($p < 0.01$) were found in women with the disease as compared to the other infertile women who were not carriers of the genotype.[2] Likewise, the iron-mediated oxidative stress that tends to cause damage of the surrounding follicles also has been found to be in association with the presence of pelvic endometriosis.

Related to the context of pelvic endometriosis, alteration of intrafollicular concentration of the proinflammatory cytokines in women with moderate/severe endometriosis undergoing ART, in comparison to the control group (tubal factor contributing to infertility) and has also been associated with maturity of the developing oocyte: FF of the follicles retrieved from women with endometriosis has shown to have a significantly higher levels of interleukin-12 and 8 in comparison to the control group, wherein the IL-8 and 12 levels were low in the FF of the follicles that contained a mature versus that of immature oocyte. Hence, the disease-related inflammatory process in FF may be contributory to the decrease in the quality of oocytes.

RECENT EVIDENCE AND META-ANALYSIS STUDIES

Recently, four meta-analyses have provided us with a clinical insight of the effects of pelvic endometriosis on the quality of the oocytes (Table 1). The first was demonstrated by Barnhart et al. in the year 2002, had put forth a comparison of the outcome of IVF in patients with endometriosis, considering the various stages of endometriosis, with patients with other causes leading to infertility (male factor, ovulatory dysfunction, and tubal factor). Overall, from the study that included database collected from 22 nonrandomized clinical trials for a total of 2,377 IVF cycles of patients with endometriosis; and 4,383 IVF cycles of unaffected patients, even when

TABLE 1: The results of the meta-analysis providing a clinical insight on the effects of pelvic endometriosis on the quality of oocytes.

		Outcome: MII oocytes retrieved		Outcome: Fertilization rate	
	Endometriosis groups (a)	*Studies included (n)*	*Endometriosis vs. controls (95% CI)*	*Studies included (n)*	*Endometriosis vs. controls (95% CI)*
Barnhart et al., 2002	Overall			Not known	Odds ratio 0.81 (0.79–0.83) (c)
	Stage I and II			Not known	Odds ratio 0.94 (0.93–0.96) (c)
	Stage III and IV			Not known	Odds ratio 1.54 (1.39–1.70) (c)
Harb et al., 2013	Untreated stage I and II			7	Relative risk 0.93 (0.87–0.99) (c)
	Untreated stage III and IV			3	Relative risk 1.01 (0.93–1.10)
Yang et al., 2015	Untreated endometriomas	2	Mean difference –3.61 (– 4.44 to – 2.78) (c)	2	Odds ratio 1.06 (0.71–1.60) (b)
Rossi et al., 2016	Overall	4	Odds ratio –1.22 – (2.38 to 0.06) (c)		
	Stage I and II	2	Odds ratio –0.55 (–1.34 to 0.25)		
	Stage III and IV	3	Odds ratio –0.83 (–1.73 to 0.08)		
	Treated with surgery	3	Odds ratio –1.62 (–3.31 to 0.07)		
	Untreated	1	Odds ratio – 0.50 (–1.59 to 0.59)		
	Endometriomas	2	Odds ratio –2.48 (–4.43 to –0.53) (c)		

(a) Where not specified, history of treatment versus untreated disease is not known (b) Control group: contralateral healthy ovary (c) statistically significant

the number of the studies included in each of the individual subanalysis groups were not reported. The adjusted analysis had noted a decrease in the rate of fertilization in women with endometriosis [Odds ratio (OR): 0.81; with a 95% confidence interval (CI): of 0.79–0.83, and p value < 0.001] in support of the deleterious impact on the quality of the oocytes. Then, the authors had separately compared the patients with minimal or mild form of the disease and those patients with moderate or severe endometriosis, with patients with tubal factor contributing to infertility. The fertilization rate in patients with severe form of the disease was much higher when compared to patients with tubal factor subfertility (OR: 1.54; with a 95%CI of 1.39–1.70, with a *p value* < 0.001), or patients with minimal or mild disease (OR: 1.11; with 95%CI of 1.09–1.13, a significant $p < 0.001$). Unfortunately, the results from this meta-analysis had not distinguished between patients who had previously received surgical and/or medical treatment, hence potentially weakening the proper source of association that had been identified.[3]

THE ESHRE GUIDELINES 2022

- For infertile patients with rASRM stage I and II endometriosis, intrauterine insemination (IUI) with ovarian stimulation can be performed, instead of considering expectant management or going for IUI alone, as it tends to increase the pregnancy rates (Omland, 1998); (Nulsen,1993); (Tummon, 1997).
- Although the success of IUI in infertile patients with rASRM stage III and IV of the disease with patent tubes may not be certain, the use of IUI along with ovarian stimulation should be put into consideration (Van der Houwen, 2014).
- IVF can be considered for subfertility associated with pelvic endometriosis, especially when there is impaired tubal function, or for male factor subfertility, and in cases with low endometriosis fertility index (EFI) or if the other treatment protocols have all failed to show results (Alshehre, 2021).
- Choosing the appropriate protocol for IVF in patients with endometriosis is challenging. Gonadotropin-releasing hormone (GnRH) agonists and antagonists can be used depending on the clinician's and the patients' preferences as there is no difference with regards to the clinical pregnancy or live birth rates (Drakopoulos et al. 2018).
- In cases of severe ovarian endometriosis, physicians may discuss with the patients the advantages and disadvantages of fertility preservation. However, the true benefits of fertility preservation for patients with endometriosis still remains to be uncertain (Kim, 2020).

EXPERIENCES OF OOCYTE DONATION

Various programs for oocyte donation have been studied recently that provides us with interesting insights regarding the causes of pelvic endometriosis and related subfertility. Of the studies that had been conducted to attain clinical-based knowledge of the main factors associated with the etiology of pelvic endometriosis and infertility was a study by Simon and coworkers as they had demonstrated that women with endometriosis almost have equal chances in relation to implantation and clinical pregnancy as with other recipients when the oocytes were retrieved from the healthy donors. However, it was reported that patients who had received embryos which were derived from the endometriotic ovaries had showed a significant reduction in the rate of implantation in comparison to the other remaining group of patients (p value < 0.05) and hence, it was hypothesized from this observation that a positive pregnancy is often related to the quality of oocytes.

Later on, the same authors have conducted a prospective study, wherein three groups were considered as for the elimination of the chances of an inherent bias which is a frequently observed nature of retrospective studies; group A patients were all the recipients and donors without the disease (n = 44); group B, consisted of donors with pelvic endometriosis who provided the oocytes to the recipients, i.e., women without the disease (n = 14) and group 3 contained the recipients and donors with the disease (n = 16). The decrease in the pregnancy rate with each transfer as noted in the group B had concluded that embryos which were derived from oocytes of patients with the disease have a lower ability of implantation owing to changes within the oocytes.

Moreover, all past studies suggest that infertility with endometriosis could not be directly linked to the endometrial environment but mostly associated with diminished quality of the oocytes. Katsoff et al. and colleagues in a recent retrospective study have failed to find differences in the pregnancy and birth rates amongst recipients who had received oocytes from healthy donors (n = 133) and (n = 21) with endometriosis; laparoscopically diagnosed. However, the calculation analysis of the study was found to be lacking and the results obtained thus were difficult to conclude.

IMPACT ON THE CLINICAL PRACTICE GUIDELINES

The are various relevant queries which may have an impact on the clinical practice guidelines which still largely remains unanswered from inconclusive studies. For instance, the extensiveness to which oocyte quality in women with pelvic endometriosis can be influenced by previous surgical/medical treatment is still difficult to determine. The only existing meta-analysis that had included the studies where women had no previous history of any surgical/medical treatments before IVF. While a reduction in the rate of fertilization for mild endometriosis has been confirmed when compared to the other causes of subfertility; unfortunately, till date the effects of endometriosis on the number of oocytes retrieved have not been evaluated as in any other meta-analyses yet. However, a very interesting recent study that included biopsies taken from the ovarian cortex in women with endometrioma and of the contralateral ovaries as derived from 13 women aged <40 years, has shown to have a significantly higher chances of oocyte apoptosis and related atresia of the follicles in the diseased ovary. More importantly, patients in the study group had relatively small endometriomas (1-4 cm, median of 2.7 cm); hence, negative effect of the early stages of the disease as per se seemed to be confirmed.[3]

The administration of a 3-6 months of GnRH agonist followed by IVF/intra-cytoplasmic sperm injection (ICSI) in women with pelvic endometriosis has previously been shown to improve clinical pregnancy rates; however, whether or not this effect was related to an ovarian or endometrial benefit still has remained uncertain as suggested by a recent Cochrane review published in the year 2006.[5] Another recent randomized controlled trial (RCT) has tested and determined the efficacy of 3-month GnRH agonist administration prior to ART, evaluating the number of MII oocytes retrieved to be the primary outcome, but has failed to find any benefit with the above. A higher dose of follicle-stimulating hormone (FSH) in the treatment protocol and longer stimulation were needed for stimulation in the group of patients with GnRH agonist used in the pretreatment phase. Moreover, women included had no history of ovarian endometriosis and were previously treated surgically for peritoneal endometriosis, and were then assigned to either as patients who underwent immediate IVF following surgery or who were subjected to GnRH agonist treatment for 3 months postsurgery and then subsequent IVF. No proper interpretation could be obtained regarding the advantages of GnRH agonist treatment for women with ovarian endometriomas or in women who had not undergone any surgical treatment for endometriosis. More relevant clinical trials are required to establish facts.

Moreover, the current evidences suggest that ICSI may be chosen over conventional IVF in women with pelvic endometriosis. A recent prospective randomized trial on women who were diagnosed laparoscopically to have moderate-severe endometriosis with normozoospermic male partners, included 786 oocytes which showed that the sibling oocytes had achieved a higher rate of fertilization with IVF/ICSI as compared to the conventional IVF cycles (73.3% vs. 54.7%, with a significant $p\ value$ < 0.01), furthermore suggesting that IVF ICSI may be the better treatment option as compared to the conventional IVF in patients with endometriosis-related subfertility.[6]

The current literature on the topic fails to provide us with any proper insight into the estimated survival rates of the frozen or thawed oocytes from patients with the disease when compared to the controls without endometriosis. Therefore, the extent of the negative effects of the disease on the quality of oocytes may also cause impairment of the proper utility of the fertility preservation techniques, and hence this option before offering to patients should be considered with caution.[3]

WHY IS IT IMPORTANT TO DO THIS REVIEW?

The long-term use of GnRH agonist prior to IVF cycles in women with endometriosis is often found to be associated with a relatively higher live birth and pregnancy rates (Sallam et al., 2006). However, live birth data was extrapolated from a single study which had reported on pregnancies that had "reached viability" (Dicker et al., 1992). Furthermore, the pregnancy rate was then calculated from meta-analysis of three other studies, of which two had reported no significant difference in their outcomes (Rickes, 2002); (Surrey, 2002), but with data reaching statistical significance owing to the size of the effect as reported by Dicker et al., 1992. Based on findings of Sallam et al., 2006, IVF/ICSI with the long-term downregulation of the pituitary has been reported to be the first choice of treatment for patients with endometriosis-related infertility **(Flowcharts 1 and 2)** (ESHRE) (2013).

Based on the data deduced from the recent studies, in women with pelvic endometriosis undergoing IVF/ICSI may be preferred over the conventional IVF; furthermore, the role of 3–6 months' use of GnRH agonists prior to commencement of treatment deserves further extensive research. Hence, the evidences in this field of study is at present far from being conclusive, particularly when considering the effect of the different stages of the disease and its relation to prior treatments on the quality of the oocyte.

To conclude, clinicians still have doubts about the effectiveness of various treatment protocols in women with endometriosis. Concerns include the possibility of having a lower response to ovarian stimulation,

Endometriosis and In Vitro Fertilization

Flowchart 1: A summary of the recent recommendations on the treatment of endometriosis-associated infertility.

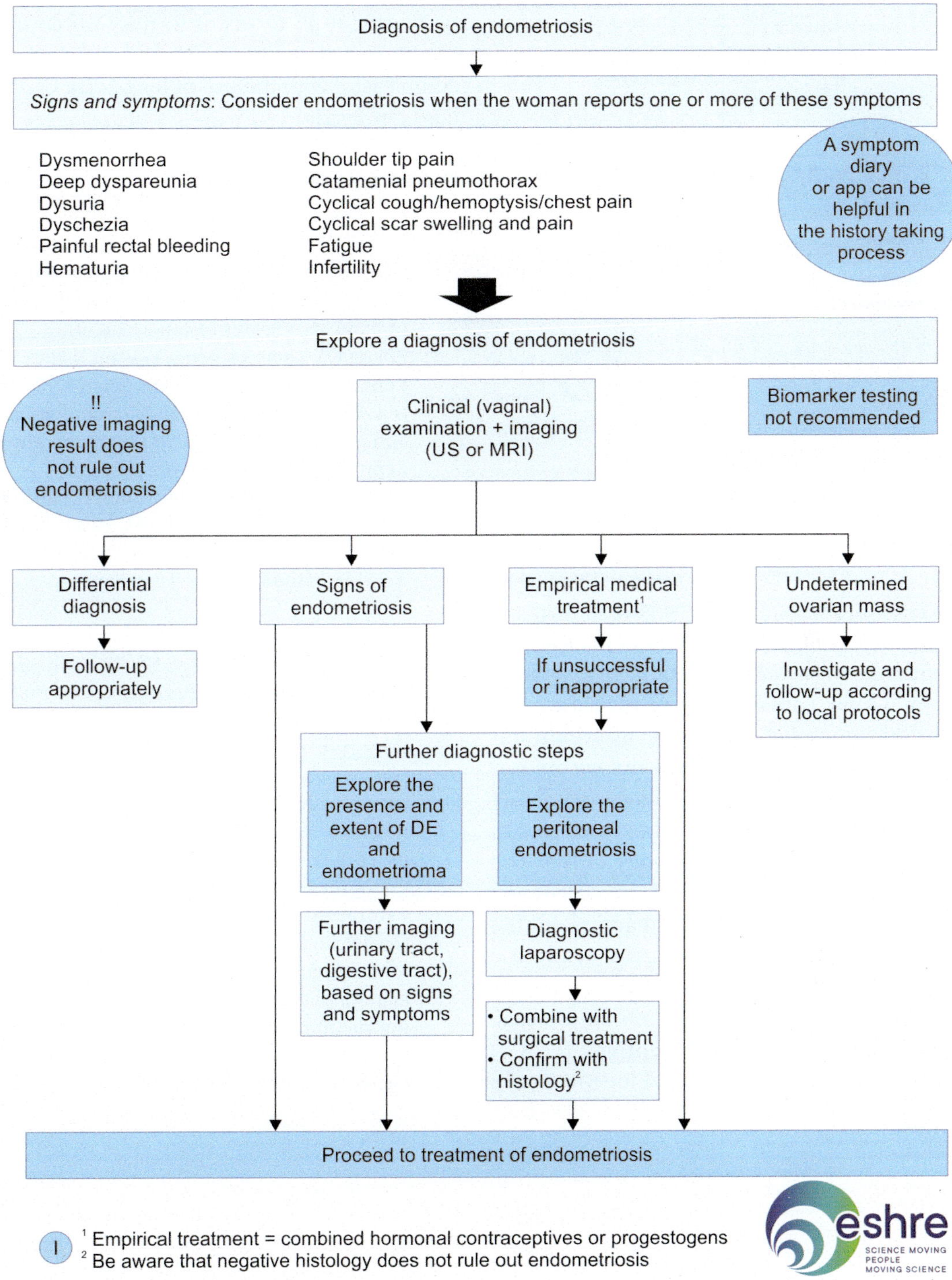

```
Diagnosis of endometriosis
            ↓
Signs and symptoms: Consider endometriosis when the woman reports one or more of these symptoms
```

- Dysmenorrhea
- Deep dyspareunia
- Dysuria
- Dyschezia
- Painful rectal bleeding
- Hematuria
- Shoulder tip pain
- Catamenial pneumothorax
- Cyclical cough/hemoptysis/chest pain
- Cyclical scar swelling and pain
- Fatigue
- Infertility

(A symptom diary or app can be helpful in the history taking process)

↓

Explore a diagnosis of endometriosis

- !! Negative imaging result does not rule out endometriosis
- Clinical (vaginal) examination + imaging (US or MRI)
- Biomarker testing not recommended

Branches:
- Differential diagnosis → Follow-up appropriately
- Signs of endometriosis
- Empirical medical treatment[1] → If unsuccessful or inappropriate
- Undetermined ovarian mass → Investigate and follow-up according to local protocols

Further diagnostic steps
- Explore the presence and extent of DE and endometrioma
- Explore the peritoneal endometriosis

- Further imaging (urinary tract, digestive tract), based on signs and symptoms
- Diagnostic laparoscopy
  - Combine with surgical treatment
  - Confirm with histology[2]

↓

Proceed to treatment of endometriosis

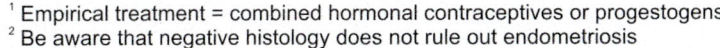
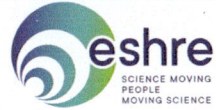

[1] Empirical treatment = combined hormonal contraceptives or progestogens
[2] Be aware that negative histology does not rule out endometriosis

Flowchart 2: Treatments for endometriosis.

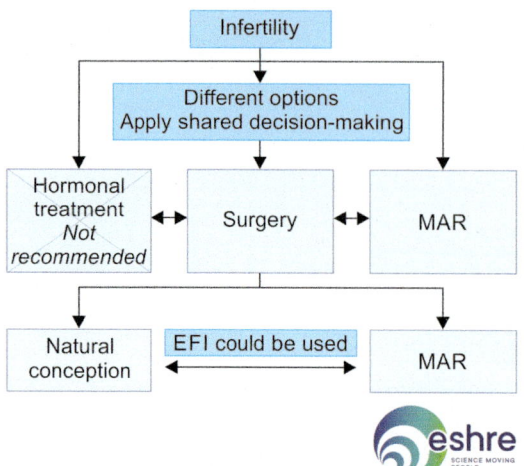

(EFI: endometriosis fertility index; MAR: medically assisted reproduction)

especially amongst the poor responders. The beneficial role and effects of the prolonged use of GnRH prior to IVF are mostly seen in cases with severe endometriosis, the benefits and harms of these intervention in mild and moderate cases have still not been evaluated fully. Other concerns focus regarding the unpleasant adverse effects of treatment with GnRH agonists such as the vasomotor symptoms and the psychological irritability of women treated with the above, which can seriously affect patient's quality of life. The complications associated with treatment are: infections, pelvic abscess formation, and the risks of ovarian hyperstimulation syndrome (OHSS), which have still not been fully assessed. Alternatively, the continuous usage of combined oral contraceptives (COCs) (have the fewest side effects) for 6–8 weeks prior to commencing IVF or ICSI in women with pelvic endometriosis has shown to be favorable in terms of fertility outcomes (de Ziegler et al. 2010), although till date no comparison with the use of long-term GnRH has been made.[5]

■ REFERENCES

1. Pop-Trajkovic S, Kopitović V, Popović J, Antić V, Radović D, Živadinović R. In vitro fertilization outcome in women with endometriosis and previous ovarian surgery. Indian J Med Res. 2014;140(3):387-91.
2. Zhang QY, Guan Q, Wang Y, Feng X, Sun W, Kong FY, et al. BDNF Val66Met polymorphism is associated with Stage III-IV endometriosis and poor in vitro fertilization outcome. Hum Reprod Oxf Engl. 2012;27(6):1668-75.
3. Sanchez AM, Vanni VS, Bartiromo L, Papaleo E, Zilberberg E, Candiani M, et al. Is the oocyte quality affected by endometriosis? A review of the literature. J Ovarian Res. 2017; 10:43.
4. Becker CM, Bokor A, Heikinheimo O, Horne A, Jansen F, Kiesel L, et al. ESHRE guideline: endometriosis. Hum Reprod Open. 2022; 2022(2):hoac009.
5. Georgiou EX, Melo P, Baker PE, Sallam HN, Arici A, Garcia-Velasco JA, et al. Long-term GnRH agonist therapy before in vitro fertilisation (IVF) for improving fertility outcomes in women with endometriosis. Cochrane Database Syst Rev. 2019;2019(11): CD013240.
6. Komsky-Elbaz A, Raziel A, Friedler S, Strassburger D, Kasterstein E, Komarovsky D, et al. Conventional IVF versus ICSI in sibling oocytes from couples with endometriosis and normozoospermic semen. J Assist Reprod Genet. 2013;30(2):251-7.

CHAPTER 12

Recurrent Endometriosis

Rohan Palshetkar, Ritu Hinduja

INTRODUCTION

Endometriosis is described by the occurrence of endometrial tissue with stroma and glands outside the uteri. Even though, a benign disease, the clinical spectrum differs extensively and is independent of the severity of the disease; pelvic endometriosis is a form of chronic inflammation. With regards to the recent available literature, the prevalence of endometriosis in patients with dysmenorrhea is found to be approaching 40–60%, whereas, in patients with infertility, it is around 20–30%. Surgery is the most widely used treatment for endometriosis; however, the significant risk of unsolved symptoms and recurrence makes endometriosis the third most common reason for hospitalization of patients worldwide.[1]

RECURRENCE RATE OF ENDOMETRIOSIS

Endometriosis is a well-defined disease entity that plays a vital role in high morbidity and contributes to high financial cost. Recurrence of the disease is frequent in women with endometriosis and ranges to a great extent among different studies. Transvaginal ultrasonography is a very sensitive and specific tool that aids clinicians in the diagnosis of endometrioma. The overall recurrence rate ranges between 6 and 68% in agreement with the different criteria that are considered clinically.

The disparity in the recurrence rate of the disease depends on various factors. Initially, the definition considered for the recurrence of endometriosis presents with dissimilarity among various studies. It may manifest as chronic pelvic pain (CPP) as reported patients (dysmenorrhea and dyspareunia) or may fulfill the clinical guiding principle of: Nodulations on imaging and examination, pelvic mass; or with persistence, in the setting of subfertility. Vignali and coworkers stated the rate of recurrence for pain after surgery in 3 and 5 years' time as 20 and 44%, respectively. The overall clinical rate of recurrence for those time intervals was 9 and 28%, respectively. Fedele et al. and coworkers reported that the rate of recurrence for dysmenorrhea was 30% after 1 year of laparoscopic surgery.

Exacoustos and colleagues phased recurrence as the presence of cysts >10 mm in diameter and stated that pelvic pain and discomfort were found to be a determinant pragmatic factor for surgical management and also that 76% of women who had recurrent endometriosis-endured pelvic pain and related symptoms. The rate of recurrence is higher for pain-related symptoms than that of clinical recurrence as identified on sonography. Also to note, the time interval for follow-up after surgical treatment as expected had an influence on the rate of recurrence. It has been recently from a meta-analysis that the 2-year rate of recurrence is 19.1%, and that of 5-year is 20.5–43.5%. Busacca and coworkers had evaluated 144 women with recurrence of the disease from 1,106 patients with pelvic endometriosis, and they reported that the 4-year rate of recurrence was 24; 30 and 23% for the superficial ovarian, deep ovarian and peritoneal endometriosis, respectively. The recurrence rate was found to increase over time after surgical treatment and the 8-year recurrence rates were 42, 24, 43, and 31%, respectively. Recently reported by Parazzini et al. that 2-year recurrence rate for stage I and II was 6%, wherein it was 14.3% for stage III/IV of the disease.[1]

RISK FACTORS FOR RECURRENT ENDOMETRIOSIS

As the various causes for recurrent endometriosis is still not clear, the revised American Fertility Society (rAFS) staging has also not been very predictive regarding the risks of recurrence (Vercellini, 2006), a great many epidemiological studies conducted worldwide for the identification of the risk factors for recurrent endometriosis.

The most commonly identified risk factors are given in the **Table 1**, based on substantial search of PUBMED.[2]

RELATIONSHIP BETWEEN PREGNANCY AND RECURRENCE

In several studies, it has been reported that pregnancy after surgical treatment acts as a factor of protection for recurrence of the disease. However, we may also state that possibly pregnancy, by itself might in fact cause suppression of inflammation and growth of the lesions owing to an elevation of the progesterone levels; another possibility is that recurrence and failure in pregnancy, either can be the failure of conception or lucidly a failure of implantation, might be solely the two-dimensional facets that usually manifest by unknown mechanisms. The two scenarios, however, represent two different dimensions for recurrence that might not be fully exclusive; and hence be delineated and distinguished in future prospective research in the field **(Fig. 1)**.[2]

RECURRENCE AND IDENTIFICATION OF BIOMARKERS

Identification of a useful tool may provide some dynamic advantages to clinicians. Firstly, establishment of the various risk factors for recurrence might help in classifying the subgroups of patients who have a significant risk, for the control of the disease. Hence, consultation with an expert surgical team or decision in accomplishing an extensive surgery may be necessary for the patients with a higher risk of recurrence. Moreover, we may not do the unnecessary interventions for the "low-profile" patients and may tailor the treatment protocol based on patient characteristics. Secondly, while establishing research about the biomarkers, the pathophysiology should be considered in details.

As endometriosis is estrogen dependent, the first class of biomarkers is associated to the mechanisms of synthesis of the sex-steroids. When we revise the basics, namely two types of estrogen receptors: Estrogen receptors alpha and beta (ER-α and β) are recognized. They comprise a DNA and an estrogen-binding domain. Subsequent to the process of binding to the ligands, the two receptors have the action similar to transcriptional factors which upregulates or downregulates the expression of the gene by their interaction with the regulatory sites of the targeted genes. With regards to the receptors,

TABLE 1: Recurrent endometriosis and the risk factors as published by recent studies.

Author and year of publication	Risk factors
Abbott et al. (2003)	rAFS > 70
Bulletti et al. (2001)	EA can be protective
Busacca et al. (1999a)	rAFS stage, previous surgery
Fedele et al. (2004)	• Younger age • Pregnancy is protective
Fedele et al. (2005)	Extent of surgical excision
Ghezzi et al. (2001)	Laterality of lesions
Jones and Sutton (2002)	Bilateral cysts
Kikuchi et al. (2006)	rAFS score, older age
Koga et al. (2006)	Previous medical treatment, size
Li et al. (2005)	• Previous surgical history, bilateral pelvic involvement, involvement of left-side pelvic, high postoperation rAFS score, younger age, painful nodule in the pouch of Douglas, use of clomifene • *Protective factors:* Number of pregnancies and postoperative progestin treatment
Liu et al. (2007)	• *For recurrence of disease:* rAFS score, younger age, previous use of medication • *For dysmenorrhea:* rAFS score
Namnoum et al. (1995)	Ovarian preservation
Parazzini et al. (2005)	rAFS stage, older age
Saleh and Tulandi (1999)	Size of the cyst
Vercellini et al. (2006)	• Younger age at surgery (for dysmenorrhea) • Postoperative medical treatment (for disease recurrence)
Vercellini et al. (2008)	OC use is a protective factor
Vignali et al. (2005)	• Younger age (for pain) • Obliteration of the Douglas pouch (for clinical signs) • Completeness of the first surgery (for reoperation)
Waller and Shaw (1993)	rAFS stage

(OC: oral contraceptive; rAFS: revised American Fertility Society)

Luisi and coworkers studied and evaluated for a possible positive correlation between *Estrogen Receptor* gene polymorphisms exist considering both the clinical and prognostic factors of recurrence of the disease. After 61 patients, with recurrence were investigated, ER-α *Pvu II* polymorphism had a frequency of PP, Pp, and pp genotypes of 55; 46 and 0%, respectively. Accordingly, patients with PP ER-α genotypes frequently had a higher bone mineral density (BMD) and a significant risk of hysterectomy at a younger age (premenopausal) due to fibroid uterus as compared to patients with other genotypes.

For the synthesis of prostaglandin, COX-2 acts as the rate-limiting enzyme and has a vital role in the overall process of proliferation and inflammatory changes of the glands related to

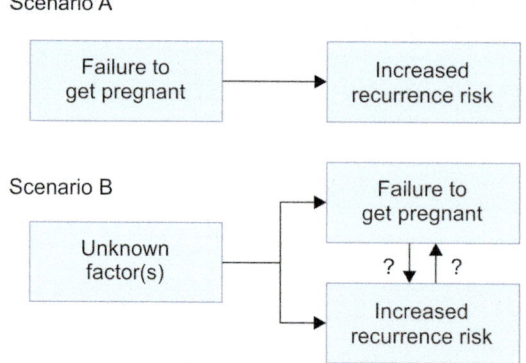

Fig. 1: The two scenarios of the relationship between clinical pregnancy and recurrent endometriosis.

the disease. Subsequently, the factors which regulate prostaglandin synthesis acts as the potential markers for predicting recurrence following surgery. Moreover, the increased expression of *COX-2* often correlates with higher incidence of dysmenorrhea, and with nonmenstrual pelvic pain in patients with the disease. Yuan and colleagues investigated 109 women for recurrent disease with histologically confirmed diagnosis from previous surgeries. The expression of *COX-2* was then evaluated by the standards of immunohistochemistry in the endometriotic tissue samples obtained, 53 women were ascertained to have recurrence and the rest of the 56 patients did not. The study demonstrated that a markedly increased level of the COX-2 scores, in the group of women with recurrent endometriosis as compared to the control group. The study reported that COX-2 enzyme overexpression may be the determining factor in women having a higher risk of recurrence. Therefore, administration of nonsteroidal anti-inflammatory drugs (NSAIDs) might be considered to be a good option for successful treatment in women with increased levels of the staining scores of the COX-2 enzyme.

The nuclear factor kappa B (NF-κB) is an important transcription factor that acts by promoting the expression of >150 genes which are involved in the cellular process including the inflammatory process, immune response, proliferation, cell adhesion, and apoptosis. The inactivation of NF-κB is by the progesterone receptors. There is always a dynamic challenge in the endometrium with the NF-κB activation and the expression of progesterone receptor-B (PR-β) Cytokines and oxidants act as the inducers for the activation of NF-κB; that leads to proliferation of endometriotic tissues. Hence, NF-κB plays a vital role in the pathophysiology of endometriosis and is a dynamic biomarker for identification of women who have significant risks of recurrence of the disease. Based on that concept, Shen et al. and coworkers had investigated 109 women having history-based confirmed endometriosis and had categorized them into groups based on presence ($n = 53$); or absence ($n = 56$) of recurrent disease, following 30 months from surgical management. The tissue blocks were stained of NF-κB p65 subunit and the progesterone receptor isoform B and the immunoreactivity of NF-κB p65 was found to be markedly high in the recurrent group of patients, and the PR-β immunoreactivity was found to be significantly higher in the nonrecurrent group of patients. In addition to the above, statistically, they had eclipsed the prediction power of COX-2 after using a regression model. Again, those findings did evoke the way of the individualized treatment modality. To cite with an example, the progestin-only treatment modalities may not be appropriate for patients having a low PR-β immunoreactivity. However, on the other side, the inhibitors of NF-κB may be more useful if there is a significant reactivity, after the histochemical staining.

RECURRENCE RISK AND THE EFFECT OF POSTOPERATIVE MEDICAL THERAPY

From various past studies, it is well ascertained that the three prime classes of medications for medical management of endometriosis includes GnRH agonists, progestins, and androgenic drugs (Danazol) cause suppression of proliferation of the implants and hence cause a reduction of adhesions (Sharpe-Timms, 1995). Therefore, medical therapy promises to be a suitable approach for the treatment of women with endometriosis in the postoperative period, with the sole purpose to eliminate the remnant endometriotic tissues and hence to diminish the risk of recurrence. Moreover, recently two expert panels have suggested that the postoperative adjuvant medical therapy should be commenced, as a way to reduce recurrence and also to increase the pain-free time interval following conservative surgical treatment, for women with stage III/IV of the disease (ACOG, 2000). Hence, a more clinically relevant question has been raised here as to ascertain if there is any form of evidence that demonstrates whether postoperative medical therapy can cause a reduction in the recurrence risk of the diseases and, if that is true, then to by what extent? However, there are major differences in the treatment modalities, the types of the disease, and the period of follow-ups and various outcome estimations that precludes any proper clinical systematic review on the topic at present.[3]

Morgante in the year 1999 stated that women treated with Danazol (100 mg/day for a period of 6 months) after surgery, and with 6 months of GnRH agonists had lesser incidence of pain in comparison to those patients who received no treatment. Especially after 2 years of laparoscopic surgery of endometriosis, 14 women received Danazol and they had a markedly lower pain score in comparison to the other group who had not received any treatment, recurrence rate, which was not very clearly outlined, was found to be 44% in the former group of patients and was 68% in the latter group of patients.

A randomized clinical trial, by Bianchi in 1999, included 77 patients with III/IV endometriosis; failed to report any statistically significant difference in the 1-year rate of recurrence amongst patients on Danazol (600 mg/day) for 3 months following surgical treatment and in those who received no treatment after surgery. The study stated that the rate of recurrence is 27 and 35%, respectively, in case group ($n = 36$), and the control group ($n = 41$).

In a multicenter, randomized, controlled study by Vercellini et al. (1999) compared the recurrence of chronic pain in patients with symptomatic disease, undergoing conservative surgical treatment and the use of GnRH agonists in the postoperative period with patients who underwent surgery alone. They reported that at the 1- and 2-year follow-ups, 14 of the 107 patients (13.1%) and 19 of 81 patients (23.5%) had moderate-to-severe symptoms pertaining to recurrence of the disease in the GnRH agonist group when in comparison with, respectively, 21.4% and 36.5% in the control group of patients ($P\ value = 0.140$ at 1 year and 0.080 at 2 years). They concluded that the postoperative treatment with GnRH agonists may significantly prolong the pain-free period after surgery, and may not have a negative influence on the reproductive health of the patients. It is not clear whether if the results, which they had ascertained on the basis of as-treated patients, should be of any difference if it was based on intent-to-treat subjects.

Muzii and co-workers in the year 2000 reported in a randomized prospective study including 70 women with III/IV endometriosis that had compared the efficacy of the postoperative medical management with low-dose oral contraceptives (OCPs) on the recurrence of the disease following laparoscopic surgery. They reported that although, the 1-year rate of recurrence was significantly low in women receiving OCPs as compared to the control group, there was no significant difference in the rate of recurrence over a 2- and 3-year period of time. It is not clear as if the no difference was genuinely owing to a lack of statistically significant conclusion in their study hypothesis.

A small randomized controlled trial by Vercellini et al. (2003b) included 20 parous patients with moderate or severe dysmenorrhea and compared the use of levonorgestrel-releasing intrauterine system (LNG-IUD) with that of no treatment for symptomatic disease after surgery. They reported a significant reduction in recurrence rate of dysmenorrhea 1 year following surgical treatment in the LNG-IUD group of patients as compared with the controls (2 in 10 or 10% vs. 9 in 20 or 45%, Odds = 0.14: 95% CI = 0.02–0.75). The proportion patients highly satisfied with treatment was more in the LNG-IUD group as compared to the control group, but the difference they reported was not of statistical significance (Odds = 3.00; with a 95% CI of 0.79–11.44). The conclusion was that the postoperative LNG-IUD usage causes reduction of the risk of recurrence of dysmenorrhea as reported in women with symptomatic disease following surgery.

Although, recent studies have failed to establish any concrete evidence with regards to the benefits of postoperative medical therapy in reducing recurrence of the disease (Liu, 2007), a retrospective, follow-up study by Vercellini in the year 2008 reported that use of OCPs markedly had reduced the risk of recurrence of the disease. They stated that women who frequently used OCPs had a risk reduction by 47% as compared to the never users. Additionally, the reduction rate also depended on the duration for which OCPs was used. This finding also appeared to be similar to a more recent study which shows the efficacy of OCPs for management of pain associated with the disease (Harada, 2007). However, caution should be taken by clinicians as the observational studies, unlike the RCTs, often include study groups as they cannot precisely eliminate biases, especially concerning that of selection of patients. Moreover, other statistical variables that can influence recurrence might not be matched properly between the groups. The administration of postoperative medical therapy might reflect on the matter that the women who used the form of medical treatment postsurgery might have been sicker than the control group, or, for the OCPs the users may have been healthier or a younger group of women than nonuser group of patients.

Another review reported that the postsurgical medical therapy with low-dose hormones for endometriosis in comparison to surgery only has not much of a benefit in relation to the outcomes of pain or clinical pregnancy rate; however, an improvement considering the disease recurrence on the basis of low rAFS score (Mean of −2.30: 95% CI of −4.03 to −0.59) (Yap, 2004). Overall, it was reported a lack of sufficient evidence reach a conclusion that use of hormonal therapy after conservative surgery for endometriosis is associated with benefits considering any of the results identified.

Clearly, the solution of these difficulties lies in designing more scientific and clinical randomized controlled trials in the future. Nevertheless, a prespecified time period for the follow-ups, usually should be no more than 2 years is ascertained and recurrence rates in the specific arms to be evaluated at the end of the study; the observations might be different if a longer time period for the follow-ups is established, even if at 2 years, there may not be much of a difference. If a study of such objectives is launched then caution should be highly taken, though. One other of the important aspects that has yet not been entirely appreciated is the increased demand for a large sample size in clinical trials. As the time for recurrence of the disease is the prime interest, the survival analysis methods might be applied for comparing the study variables with regards to the cause–effect recurrence rates. For detection of a 20% rate reduction with a power of the study 80% and a type I error of 5%; application of standardized measurements (Schoenfeld, 1981) indicated that 650 recurrences need to be reported in studies. Therefore, pertaining to the huge undertakings required, which would need vast resources and a large patient database that a very few medical institutions can offer independently research becomes a challenge.

Even if the postoperative medical therapy does prove to be an effective modality to reduce the recurrence risk of endometriosis, it is still questionable whether if "all" patients would be requiring medications to reduce the recurrence risk. It has been stated that 9% of patients with pelvic endometriosis have no response to progestin therapy, which may be a result of PR-β downregulation. If the PR-β is silenced due to the promoter methylation, as seen in endometriosis, treatment with progestin or OCPs may be of no value as the action of progestin is mainly through PR-β.

Hence, use of postoperative medical therapy might cause adverse effects (and also higher healthcare expenses) in some women who might intrinsically have a lesser risk than the others and in those who might simply be resistant to therapy. The identification of the high-risk individuals who might benefit from interventions would still remain as a dispute to resolve. Lastly, whether the use of a single medication would be considered to be the optimal intervention as an option is still unknown. The recent findings report that PR-β and NF-κB together may act as the primary biomarkers for recurrent disease, and also on the possibility that may be combination of drugs be the better option to the use of a single drug in risk reduction, especially if the PR-β is silenced by methylation of promotor.

■ EXECUTIVE SUMMARY

- In practice, it is very difficult to eliminate the risks of recurrence completely, after treatment of the disease.
- Numerous risk factors have been reported in the recent, and they could be classified on an individual basis or pertaining to the disease and also on the surgery-determining factors.
- As an extensive surgical treatment by a skilled surgeon team usually reduces the risks, patient and the disease-related high-risk factors stay enigmatic.
- Recent studies report that oral contraceptive pills (OCPs) have diminished the risk of recurrence of endometriosis post-surgery.
- The approach made toward finding a specific biomarker for recurrence should not only lead to the emergence of an individualized treatment protocol, but also might make clinicians decipher better the pathology pertaining to the

disease and isolate as much as possible the factors related to endometriosis and recurrence.
- At present, COX-2 enzyme and NF-κB transcription factor are the two important markers for recurrence. However, the clinical and scientific data are scarce and more specialized trials with the focus on the recurrence of the disease is urgently needed.[4]

■ CONCLUSION

To conclude, it is evident that despite the numerous attempts in the field of exploration of the risk factors, the chances of elimination of the odds which stand with regards to recurrence is still not optimistic. There is an urgent need to establish patient based individualized risk factors and the biomarkers may be the tool for future prediction of the disease. After application of the same strategy, a novel targeted and an individualized treatment modality could be explored and used in accordance to the patient characteristics.

■ REFERENCES

1. Selçuk İ, Bozdağ G. Recurrence of endometriosis; risk factors, mechanisms and biomarkers; review of the literature. J Turk Ger Gynecol Assoc. 2013;14(2):98-103.
2. Guo SW. Recurrence of endometriosis and its control. Hum Reprod Update. 2009;15(4):441-61.
3. Choi SH, Kim SE, Lim HH, Lee DY, Choi D. Efficacy of Post-Operative Medication to Prevent Recurrence of Endometrioma: Cyclic Oral Contraceptive (OC) After Gonadotropin-Releasing Hormone (GnRH) Agonist Versus Dienogest. J Korean Med Sci. 2022;37(26):e207.
4. Ceccaroni M, Bounous VE, Clarizia R, Mautone D, Mabrouk M. Recurrent endometriosis: a battle against an unknown enemy. Eur J Contracept Reprod Health Care. 2019;24(6):464-74.

Index

Page numbers followed by *f* refer to figure, *fc* refer to flowchart, and *t* refer to table

A

Adnexa 30
American Association of
    Gynecologic
    Laparoscopists 6, 24
  classification 12, 12*f*
American Society for
    Reproductive Medicine
    7, 8*t*, 16, 21, 21*f*, 44,
    60, 68
  revised classification of
    endometriosis 7, 8*t*
Angiogenesis 18
Anti-Müllerian hormone 53
Aromatase inhibitors 37, 51
Assisted reproductive technology
    44, 47, 60, 68
  indications for 54
Atorvastatin 58
Autoantibodies 18

B

Bladder 24, 30
  anterior compartments of 32*f*
  endometriosis 16
  posterior compartments
    of 32*f*
Blood biomarkers 18
Bone mineral density 77
Bowel 30
Brain-derived neurotrophic
    factor 68

C

Cabergoline 38, 58
Cancer
  antigen 3, 18
  benign 1
  ovarian 1, 2*fc*
Cervix 30
Clomiphene citrate 62, 63, 63*t*,
    64, 65
Coelomic metaplasia 7

Computed tomography scan 20
Conservative surgery,
    outcomes of 42
Controlled ovarian
    hyperstimulation 60
    stimulation 61
C-reactive protein 18
Cyst, endometriotic 19*f*, 20*f*
Cystectomy 41
  laparoscopic 52
Cytokines, inflammatory 18

D

Danazol 37, 51
Deep infiltrating endometriosis
    15, 26, 29, 52*f*, 53
  Enzian classification of 27*f*
Deoxyribonucleic acid 1
Diarrhea 47
Dienogest 51
Douglas pouch 17, 29, 30
Dyschezia 28, 47
Dysmenorrhea 28, 47, 75
Dyspareunia 28, 47, 75
Dysuria 28, 47

E

Embryo transfer 67
Endocrine abnormalities 47
Endometrial stromal tissue 19
Endometrioma 15, 21, 30, 52*f*
Endometriosis 1, 2*fc*, 6, 12*f*, 15,
    17, 24, 25*f*, 36, 44, 47,
    48*f*, 52, 53, 57, 58, 60, 67,
    68*f*, 69, 75
  bowel deep infiltrating 33*f*
  classification for 47, 49*f*
  deep 7, 24, 28, 41
    infiltrating 15, 26, 29,
      52*f*, 53
  development 45
  diagnosis of 17, 22, 24

enigma 1
Enzian classification of 11*f*
epidemiology of 46*f*
fertility index 7, 26, 48, 70, 74
    classification 9*t*, 10*t*
lesions, evolution of 2*fc*
malignant transformation
    of 1
medical management of 36
mild 60, 63
mild to moderate 61*f*
minimal 60, 63
moderate 60
ovarian 7, 24, 41
pathogenesis of 45, 45*f*
pelvic 67
peritoneal 41
premenarchal 6
recurrent 75, 76, 77*t*, 78*f*
Research Foundation 27*f*
revised classification
    of 21*f*, 25*f*
scoring systems 24
severe 60
staging for 47, 49*f*
superficial 24, 28, 52*f*
surgical management of 40
symptoms of 47, 47*t*
therapy 51
treatments for 74*fc*
Endometrium 47, 62
Enzian classification 7, 11*f*, 12,
    26, 27*f*
  revised 9
Epiphenomenon 1
Epithelial cells 57
Estradiol 63
Estrogen receptor 77
European Society for
    Gynaecological
    Endoscopy 6, 24
European Society of Human
    Reproduction and
    Embryology 6, 17, 24,
    41, 44, 60
  guidelines 70

Index

F

Federation of Obstetric and Gynaecological Societies of India 44
Fibroblast growth factor-2 188
Follicle-stimulating hormone 62-64, 71
Follicular fluid 68
Follistatin 18
Frozen embryo transfer 53

G

Genetics 7
Glycodelin A 18
Glycoproteins 18
Gonadotropin-releasing hormone 38, 41, 70
  agonists 37, 51, 61
  antagonists 38

H

Hematochezia 28, 47
Hematuria 28
  macroscopic 47
  microscopic 47
Heme 1
Hemoglobin, extracellular 1
Hepatocyte
  growth factor 18
  nuclear factor 1-beta 2
Human chorionic gonadotropin 61
Human endometrial stromal cells 58
Human menopausal gonadotropin 62, 64
Hysterectomy 42

I

In vitro fertilization 26, 52, 62, 67
Infertility 47, 60
  endometriosis-related 48
  male 54
Inflammatory disease 6
International deep endometriosis analysis 28
International ovarian tumor analysis 29, 30
Intracytoplasmic sperm injection 71

Intrauterine insemination 53, 60, 63
  clinical impact 65
  protocols 60
Iron 1

K

Kirsten rat sarcoma viral oncogene homolog 2

L

Laparoscopic uterine nerve ablation 42
Laparoscopy 20, 28
  surgery 40
Lesions, endometriotic 15
Letrozole 62, 63t
Leuprolide acetate 37
Levonorgestrel-releasing intrauterine system 80
Lovastatin 58
Luteinizing hormone 61, 63, 68

M

Magnetic resonance imaging 19, 26
Malignancy, endometriosis-associated 1
Malignant transformation
  early detection of 3
  mechanism of 1, 2fc
Matrix metalloproteinases 46
Menstrual pain, severe 47
Menstrual stem cells 57
Mesenchymal epithelial transition factor 2
Microembolization 6
Mifepristone 37
Monocyte chemoattractant protein-1 18
Morphological uterus sonographic assessment 30
Multidetector computerized tomography enema 26

N

Nafarelin 37
National Institute for Health and Care Excellence 61

Nonsteroidal anti-inflammatory drugs 37, 78
Nuclear factor kappa B 46

O

Oocyte
  donation 70
  quality of 69t
Oophorectomy 42
Oral contraceptive
  combined 36, 51, 74
  low-dose 80
  pills 77, 81
Ovarian cancer pathogenesis, endometriosis-associated 2fc
Ovarian clear cell cancer 3
Ovarian endometrioma 15, 28, 29, 41, 52
  size of 30
Ovarian endometriosis 7, 24, 41
  cysts 21
Ovarian hyperstimulation syndrome 65, 74
Ovarian masses 30
Ovarian suppression 51
Ovulatory dysfunction 69

P

Pelvic adhesions 20f
Pelvic nerve pathways, interruption of 42
Pelvic pain, chronic 28, 47, 75
Phosphatidylinositol-4, 5-bisphosphate 3-kinase catalytic subunit alpha 2
Platelet-derived growth factor 18
Pollakiuria 47
Pregnancy 76
Presacral neurectomy 42
Progesterone-containing contraceptives 36
Progestins 51
Proteomics 19

R

Radical surgery 42
Randomized controlled trial 51, 71
Rapamycin, mammalian target of 2

Index

Reactive oxygen species 46
Rectosigmoid junction 30, 31
Rectovaginal nodules 31
Rectovaginal septum 9, 30, 31
Rectum 24, 30, 31
Retrograde menstruation, Sampson's theory of 6
Revised American Society for Reproductive Medicine 7, 26
    classification 7

S

Sampson's theory 6
Selective estrogen receptor modulators 51
Selective progesterone receptor modulators 37
Sigmoid 31
    colon 30
Simvastatin 58
Society of Obstetricians and Gynaecologists of Canada 44
Soluble epidermal growth factor 18
Sorafenib 58
Stem cell 3, 57, 58
    therapy 57, 58
Steroidogenesis 67
Superficial peritoneal lesions 15
Superovulation 53

T

Tenesmus 47
Transvaginal scan 19
Transvaginal sonography 26
Tubal factor 69
Tuboovarian complex 10
Tumor necrosis factor alpha 46, 60

U

Ulipristal acetate 37
Ultrasound 19
Ureteric lesions 41
Ureters 30
Urine biomarkers 19
Uterine adenomyosis 16
Uterosacral ligaments 24, 30, 31
Uterovesical region 30
Uterus 30, 57
    anteverted 31f
    retroverted 31f

V

Vagina 24
Vaginal fornix, posterior 30
Vaginal septum 9
Vaginal wall 31
Vascular endothelial growth factor 18, 46, 60

W

World Endometriosis Society 24, 44

Z

Zona pellucida 68f